Positive Options for Living with Lupus

About the Author

Philippa Pigache has been a journalist and writer for more than thirty years, has written for local and national newspapers, women's magazines, radio, and television, and is currently a freelance medical science writer. She has contributed for twenty years to consumer health pages and to journals for health professionals and has won awards both for her medical journalism and for her fiction. She is currently the honorary secretary of the Medical Journalists' Association and editor of their journal, the *MJA News*.

She has written consumer health books on arthritis and attention deficit hyperactivity disorder (ADHD). Her first book, *Living with Rheumatoid Arthritis*, was commended in the 2005 MJA Open Consumer Book Awards. She has two children, three grandchildren, and three cats, lives in Sussex, England, and paints and gardens in her spare time.

Titles in the Positive Options for Health series

Positive Options for Antiphospholipid Syndrome (APS)
by Triona Holden

Positive Options for Children with Asthma by O. P. Jaggi, M.D., Ph.D.

Positive Options for Colorectal Cancer by Carol Ann Larson

Positive Options for Crohn's Disease by Joan Gomez, M.D.

Positive Options for Hiatus Hernia by Tom Smith, M.D.

Positive Options for Living with Your Ostomy by Dr. Craig A. White

Positive Options for Polycystic Ovary Syndrome (PCOS)
by Christine Craggs-Hinton & Adam Balen, M.D.

Positive Options for Reflex Sympathetic Dystrophy (RSD) by Elena Juris

Positive Options for Seasonal Affective Disorder (SAD)
by Fiona Marshall & Peter Cheevers

Positive Options for Sjögren's Syndrome by Sue Dyson

Positive Options for Living with Lupus by Philippa Pigache

Ordering

Trade bookstores in the U.S. and Canada please contact:

Publishers Group West
1700 Fourth Street, Berkeley CA 94710
Phone: (800) 788-3123   Fax: (510) 528-3444

Hunter House books are available at bulk discounts for textbook course
adoptions; to qualifying community, health-care, and government
organizations; and for special promotions and fund-raising.
For details please contact:

Special Sales Department
Hunter House Inc., PO Box 2914, Alameda CA 94501-0914
Phone: (510) 865-5282   Fax: (510) 865-4295
E-mail: ordering@hunterhouse.com

Individuals can order our books from most bookstores, by calling
(800) 266-5592, or from our website at www.hunterhouse.com

Project Credits

Cover Design:	Brian Dittmar Graphic Design
Book Production:	Hunter House
Copy Editor:	Kelley Blewster
Proofreader:	Herman Leung
Indexer:	Candace Hyatt
Acquisitions Editor:	Jeanne Brondino
Editor:	Alexandra Mummery
Publishing Interns:	Blair Cavagrotti, Faith Merino
Customer Service Manager:	Christina Sverdrup
Order Fulfillment:	Washul Lakdhon
Administrator:	Theresa Nelson
Computer Support:	Peter Eichelberger
Publisher:	Kiran S. Rana

Positive Options

for

Living with Lupus

Self-Help and Treatment

Philippa Pigache

Hunter House Inc., Publishers
PO Box 2914
Alameda CA 94501-0914

Library of Congress Cataloging-in-Publication Data

Pigache, Philippa.
Positive options for living with lupus : self-help and treatment / Philippa Pigache.
p. cm. — (Positive options for health series)
"First published as Living with lupus in Great Britain in 2005 by Sheldon Press."
Includes index.
ISBN-13: 978-0-89793-487-9
ISBN-10: 0-89793-487-3
1. Systemic lupus erythematosus—Alternative treatment. 2. Self-help techniques. I. Title.
RC924.5.L85P54 2006
616.7'7206—dc22   2006020290

Printed and Bound by Bang Printing, Brainerd, Minnesota

Manufactured in the United States of America

9 8 7 6 5 4 3 2   First Edition   07 08 09 10

Contents

DEDICATION

To my colleague and friend Tom Smith, who
held my hand on the wolf hunt.

▶ ▶ ▶

Introduction

What is lupus? Ask the medical experts and they will tell you that it is an *autoimmune disease*. Its full name is *systemic lupus erythematosus*, or SLE, though we will be referring to it as "lupus" for short. The "systemic" indicates that it affects many organs—the whole system. The "erythematosus," from the Greek word for "red," describes a certain kind of rash and refers to the part of the body most noticeably affected in lupus: the skin. Until the nineteenth century, lupus was thought of only as a skin disease. In fact, the name was almost certainly applied to other diseases affecting the skin on the face, not to what we know as lupus today.

"Lupus" is Latin for "wolf." The name of the disease was coined seven centuries ago by medieval physicians Rogerius and Paracelsus to describe facial lesions that ate into the skin and looked like a wolf bite. These days, doctors think it more likely that such lesions were caused by a form of tuberculosis rather than by what we now call lupus. In the past SLE was also sometimes called lupus vulgaris, or common lupus. This was to distinguish it from a slightly different kind of rash: discoid lupus, so called because its main symptom was raised circular discs. It is now considered to be a different version of SLE.

For the moment forget about the wolf. Think instead of the butterfly, a word used to describe a rash that appears on the faces of many people with lupus. It fans out from the bridge of the nose across the cheeks and ranges in color from rose pink to angry red.

The fact that lupus affected other organs besides the skin was not understood until the end of the nineteenth century, when it was discovered that lupus involved inflammation of the joints (*arthritis*), fatigue, and a number of other physical symptoms, including potentially fatal kidney damage. Once the link between the skin rash and fatal kidney disease had been established, lupus got very bad press. Medical textbooks printed in the first half of the twentieth century spoke of it with gloom and despondency. Ninety percent of sufferers are women of childbearing age, so female lupus sufferers were warned against getting pregnant or going out in the sun (lupus can increase the skin's sensitivity to sunlight). Sadly, a few medical professionals still cleave to this opinion. If you or someone you love has lupus, I am pleased to inform you that this is old-fashioned rubbish. Before refined laboratory tests were developed to identify the condition, the only recognized cases were people who had a severe case of the disease and had remained untreated for many years. Now that lupus is more readily diagnosed and treated, it has been established that many people have it, but only quite mildly. In fact the current belief is that there are thousands of "sleeping" lupus sufferers who go peacefully to their graves for some quite unrelated cause, unaware that they ever had the illness.

Those whose condition is diagnosed cannot yet be offered a cure, but increased understanding of what goes on in the disease, combined with modern treatment, takes the bite out of lupus. The wolf may not be dying out, but it is certainly a much less threatening creature than thought to be in the past.

Nevertheless, lupus is still a mysterious illness. Like its namesake, it lurks in the shadows of the forest and comes out at night to leave unexplained damage and devastation. And, like the animal in the fable wearing sheep's clothing, it is difficult to recognize and often gets mistaken for something else. My hope is that this book will explain some of the mysteries surrounding lupus.

Hints for the Reader

You can read this book from beginning to end, or simply dip in and out, picking out what interests or concerns you. Only the first two chapters, which explain the key features of lupus, are essential to understanding the rest of the book. Chapters 4 and 5, on diagnosis, are important if you think that you, or someone close to you, may be a sufferer. Chapters 6, 7, and 8, on treatment and management, are important for someone already confirmed with lupus. I have tried to use titles and subheads that will help you find what you are in search of. You can also refer to the Index.

Difficult words are explained in the text. Those printed in *italic type* when they first appear are also listed in the Glossary, located at the end of the book. Some interesting information on the general story of lupus is separated out in boxes.

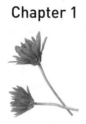

Chapter 1

Recognizing Lupus

First thing in the morning you peer into the mirror and notice a bright-red rash. From the bridge of your nose it spreads in the shape of a butterfly across both cheeks. If you had spent the previous day unprotected in bright sunlight, you might wonder if you had a sunburn, but most probably you would think, "Heavens! I've caught something. Was it something I ate?"

That's the thing about skin. It is the largest organ of the body and, being on the outside, it is extremely noticeable. As teenagers we subjected every pimple, lump, or blemish to minute examination, and each one filled us with anxiety. As adults we learn to take the odd spot, bruise, or wrinkle in stride, but a rash is different. Perhaps it is our recollection of childhood ailments such as measles or chickenpox; perhaps it is the association between rash and eating or touching something dangerous; perhaps it is even a dim folk memory of historic but fatal epidemics like smallpox or the plague. Either way, we know, almost instinctively, that a rash is a sign of something wrong. If it's on your face you can't ignore it. If it sticks around for some days you will almost certainly take it to the doctor.

This is why the oldest recognized symptom of lupus is a rash. Other symptoms may be explained away, ignored, or not recognized as being part of an illness, but a rash on the face merits attention.

The Multiple Personalities of Lupus

Like the butterfly, lupus has more than one incarnation. Suppose that instead of a rash you wake in the morning with inexplicable fever, headache, or fatigue. Suppose every joint and muscle in your body seems to ache. Suppose your eyes are dry and scratchy or your hair comes out in clumps on your comb. Suppose your ankles get puffy, or that you become so depressed you feel life is hardly worth living. Would you conclude that you had something serious? Would you think it worth bothering the doctor about? Or would you decide that you were a bit run down or starting a cold, and take a few days off in the hope that it might all blow over?

This is why the multiple manifestations of lupus took so long to become recognized. Lupus is systemic—that is, it affects many organs throughout the body—and lupus is *chronic:* It comes and goes. Left untreated it may afflict you for days or weeks but then may inexplicably clear up and leave you in peace for months or even years. At first there is no permanent damage; your body temperature goes down, your skin clears, the aches and pains go away, and your hair grows back in. There may be clues that all is not well—the rash may flare up if you are out in the sun; other symptoms may recur if you eat certain foods or go through a period of stress. You begin to notice that your body has started reacting to things that didn't bother it before. But it is perfectly possible to live with the wolf known as lupus for years without being aware of it.

By describing it as chronic and systemic we explain when and where lupus occurs. By classifying it as an autoimmune disease we indicate which bodily system underlies what goes wrong in lupus. We will explore this in more detail in Chapter 3. Put simply, in lupus, *antibodies,* which are part of the body's defense system that are normally produced to ward off foreign invaders like bacteria or viruses, start misbehaving and attack the body's own tissues.

There are other diseases in which the body's defense system runs amok; most of these conditions have only recently begun to be understood, and even then imperfectly. The best known is type 1 diabetes, in which part of the immune system destroys the cells that manufacture insulin, a hormone the body needs in order to break down the sugars in food to supply energy. Autoimmune cells are also involved in some cancers, such as *leukemia*. More significantly for people with lupus, they are implicated in *rheumatoid arthritis*, a disease closely related to lupus and sometimes mistaken for it.

Relatives of Lupus

Once you know which family lupus comes from, and who some of its close relatives are, it becomes easier to understand why it is so easily mistaken for other, similar diseases. Lupus forms part of a big family called *connective tissue diseases:* CTD for short. Connective tissue is present all over the body, which is why the symptoms of lupus are so diffuse. It includes skin, as well as the lining or sheath of joints, tendons, ligaments, blood vessels, nerves, and major organs like the heart and lungs. Arthritis, the name for conditions that affect joints (*arthros* is Greek for "joint"), is the best-known member of the CTD family. There are over one hundred forms of arthritis alone, so they might better be known in the plural as arthri*tes*. Other CTDs include systemic *sclerosis* (from the Greek word for "hardening"), which affects skin and connective tissue all over the body; *polymyositis* and *dermatomyositis* (from the Greek *myo*, for "muscle," and *derma*, for "skin"), also called PM-DM, which involves the inflammation of various muscles; plus a host of other rare disorders and syndromes. We will look at them in more detail in Chapter 9. Some CTDs defy any of the established labels; doctors call them "mixed connective tissue diseases" or MCTDs.

It's all very confusing. That's because connective tissue is ubiquitous—found all over the body—which means not only that it can give rise to a vast range of symptoms, but also that there is a wide overlap of symptoms among CTDs. North American and European medical institutions have made some progress toward inscribing diagnostic criteria in stone, but ultimately the naming of diseases is an imperfect science. In many cases uncertainty prevails, a situation that proves frustrating for both patient and doctor.

It may seem pointless or frivolous to waste time and effort over precise medical labeling (what doctors refer to as establishing a *differential diagnosis*). But it plays a vital role in deciding what treatment is likely to work and what outcome to expect.

Medical Specialists Who Treat Lupus

Because lupus affects so many different parts of the body, a patient can come into contact with a vast array of medical specialists. Immunologists specialize in the immune system. Dermatologists treat skin diseases. Rheumatologists specialize in diseases that cause inflammation (lupus is a form of arthritis caused by inflammation). An ophthalmologist, a specialist in conditions of the eye, may be consulted if the eyes are affected. A nephrologist, a kidney specialist, may also be consulted, because in its worst manifestations lupus can damage the kidneys. If the disease affects the membranes that enclose the heart or lungs, a cardiologist may be consulted. If a lupus sufferer becomes pregnant she may develop a blood disorder and need to consult a hematologist (*hem-* is from the Greek for "blood"). Many lucky lupus sufferers never get referred to specialists but instead remain in the care of their family doctor; even they will need the services of a pathologist, who specializes in analyzing the sophisticated laboratory tests that tell you what's wrong and how treatment is progressing.

Presenting Symptoms: The Patient's View

There are two ways of considering symptoms: the patient's view and the doctor's. They obviously overlap, but their significance is viewed differently. The patient has the intimate, day-to-day experience of living in his or her body. Some days feel better than others, and there are all sorts of minor aches, pains, bumps, or blemishes that come and go, signifying nothing. How a person reacts to them depends somewhat on whether he or she is a bit of a hypochondriac or tends to keep a stiff upper lip about things.

Doctors know this and do their best to make allowances for it. They figure out that Mrs. Smith thinks she has developed an allergy every time she has a touch of indigestion, whereas they don't see poor old Mr. Thomas until he has taken to his bed with pneumonia. But the patient's variable response to illness is a particular problem for doctors when the disease in question slips in and out of the forest every now and then leaving almost no trail, like lupus.

Janet's Story

Janet discovered she had lupus in 1978, when she became pregnant. She was in her late twenties. "You name a complication of pregnancy, and I had it," she says. "Blood clots, raised blood pressure, edema [puffiness caused by fluid retention] up to my knees. And then a blood clot started blocking my heart. My obstetrician said I was lucky to have survived the pregnancy and that I should not risk another one."

Fortunately he also asked Janet several probing questions and discovered that as a teenager she had suffered from a short attack of painfully swollen hands. Her doctor had put it down to rheumatoid arthritis. She also told her obstetrician that she had developed curious lumps in her legs when she had taken the birth control pill. The obstetrician said she might have "collagen disease" and recommended that she see a rheumatologist. Janet was fortunate that by then laboratory tests had been developed that provided a more conclusive diagnosis than the one offered by the shifting kaleidoscope of symptoms found with CTDs. Systemic lupus was diagnosed, and by the time Janet was ready to undertake another pregnancy her doctors made sure she received treatment that prevented all the previous complications.

Let us look at lupus symptoms as the patient experiences them:

Malaise

"Malaise" is a French word for feeling generally unwell and uncomfortable. It has that "can't-put-your-finger-on-it" character that makes it likely to be overlooked as a significant symptom of real illness. It may be accompanied by a slightly raised temperature or a headache. Malaise, with or without fever, is the most common feature of lupus and probably, when the patient looks back, the first he or she experienced, though the patient didn't identify it at the time.

It is most likely caused by the disseminated (widespread or systemic) nature of lupus. Connective tissues all over the body may be inflamed—some in the joints, others in the brain—which can lead to headaches or depression. Furthermore, a lupus sufferer may be anemic, meaning that the supply of important oxygen- and glucose-carrying red cells in the blood is depleted, a condition that causes feelings of malaise. If a person goes to the doctor with these symptoms, lupus as a cause can be easily missed or mislabeled as "post-viral fatigue," fibromyalgia, or infectious mononucleosis ("glandular fever").

Skin Rash

Only about a fifth of those with lupus experience the classic butterfly rash as their first symptom. Ultimately about half have it. Nevertheless, the skin is one of the organs most commonly involved in the illness. The rash doesn't hurt or itch, though it may burn slightly if exposed to sunlight. In fact, the lupus rash is a bit of a werewolf. It takes several forms and appears in diverse places. It is sometimes faint and rosy and, because it often follows exposure to ultraviolet light, can occasionally be mistaken for sunburn. Other times it takes the form of disc-shaped, scaly, red patches, which can appear anywhere on the body and can leave scars when they clear up. They can occur in the scalp, causing hair loss that may be permanent. (Hair loss, which strictly speaking is another skin symptom, may occur even in the absence of a rash. On those occasions it invariably regrows.) These raised plaques are the discoid lesions that occur in about 15 percent of lupus sufferers, the vast majority of whom have none of the other lupus symptoms. For this reason, in the past, this skin condition was often classified as a separate illness, discoid lupus erythematosus. Because their symptoms are so mild, it is likely that patients with discoid lesions slip between the population statistics of lupus; in many parts of the world they may not even consult a doctor for their symptoms.

Sometimes the rash takes the form of small blisters (*vesicles*), which are caused by inflammation in the small blood vessels. These may appear on the face, neck, elbows, palms, tips of the fingers, or soles of the feet. Blisters on the feet can easily be missed unless there are accompanying symptoms. Vesicles can also crop up on the mouth in the form of painless ulcers, and occasionally in the vagina. About one in eight lupus patients has these blisters at some time or other.

Faced with any of these types of rashes, a doctor is on much firmer ground than with malaise. Lupus will definitely be among his or her likely suspects.

Before we leave the topic of the skin manifestations of lupus, it is worth mentioning a very common symptom: About a third of lupus patients are *photosensitive*—that is, they react in an extreme way to ultraviolet light, with inflammation, burning, and blistering. Some also react to fluorescent lights. In terms of diagnosis, this symptom has the advantage of being closely associated with lupus but with few other CTDs.

Arthritis

As we saw in Janet's case, lupus is easily mistaken for rheumatoid arthritis. In both illnesses the joints most commonly affected are those of the hands, arms, feet, and legs. Joint pain is the first-noted symptom in about three-quarters of lupus cases, and over 90 percent of diagnosed cases experience arthritis at some time. The most common pattern is to experience stiffness, tenderness, and swelling of the fingers and wrists upon waking. Unlike the joint pain in rheumatoid arthritis, which in many cases is unremitting unless treated, lupus arthritis usually comes and goes and varies in intensity.

Shannon's Story

Shannon worked in a busy insurance office and spent most of her time at the computer keyboard. She was thirty-three when she first noticed signs of arthritis—stiffness, swelling, and pain— in her hands. "It's a bit early for osteoarthritis," she said to herself. (Osteoarthritis is not caused by inflammation but mostly by normal wear and tear and doesn't usually show up until someone is in their fifties.) She also wondered about repetitive strain injury or carpal tunnel syndrome, two conditions that often bother people who type a lot. She took acetominophen and tried to ignore it. But then she and her husband went on a walking vacation over a three-day weekend. "On the first day we must have covered ten or fifteen miles, a distance we could usually handle easily," she said. "But the following morning I just couldn't get out of bed. The weekend was ruined. The pain continued into the week. I couldn't go to work and ended up lying in bed with packs of frozen peas on my knees and ankles, unable to get up or go to sleep." Shanon's husband called the doctor, who thought it was probably rheumatoid arthritis. But when the doctor asked about Shannon's medical history Shannon remembered that she'd had mouth ulcers a few years back. The doctor sent samples of Shannon's blood to the laboratory. The results confirmed that it was lupus.

Heart and Lung Problems

The heart and lungs are both surrounded by membranes made of connective tissue. The heart membrane is called the *pericardium;* inflammation of the pericardium is called *pericarditis.* The membranes enclosing the lungs are called the *pleura;* inflammation of the pleura is *pleurisy.* When these membranes become inflamed the patient experiences pain, especially during breathing. These symptoms are unlikely to be the first ones experienced by anyone with lupus, but if a patient has fever and malaise that he or she attributes to flu or a bad cold, the condition may escalate to bronchitis, pneumonia, and then pleurisy. If things get to this stage the person will almost certainly be admitted to the hospital. Lots of tests will be done to identify the problem, resulting ultimately in an accurate diagnosis, even if a number of others are considered first. As one patient put it, "There isn't a single test that says unequivocally, 'Yes, you have lupus.' You sort of back into it after visiting several other possibilities." Studies show that between 33 and 45 percent of lupus sufferers have pleurisy at some time or another, and about 25 percent may develop pericarditis.

Kidney Problems

Half of lupus sufferers develop some degree of kidney involvement. These symptoms, although unlikely to be among the first encountered by someone with lupus, can have a potentially fatal outcome. Prior to the 1940s, before modern understanding of the disease and modern drugs to treat it, it was kidney failure that gave lupus such a bad name.

Kidney problems first manifest in the form of puffy ankles and possibly puffy fingers and knees. When the kidneys are unable to adequately filter waste products from the body, fluid builds up, starting in the ankles and working its way up (due to gravity). When fluid remains pooled in the tissues it causes swelling and discomfort called *edema*. Edema is easy to identify because if you press a finger into the swelling the indentation does not fade for some minutes. Edema is a signal that the kidneys are not functioning. It is quite common in the latter stages of pregnancy, even for women without lupus. It is confirmed by a simple urine test that detects the presence of protein fragments normally filtered out of the urine by healthy kidneys.

Blood Problems

I have already mentioned that the malaise associated with lupus can partly be attributed to a shortage of red blood cells, a condition known as anemia. Supplies of other blood cells may also be affected, including white cells, which fight off disease, and platelets, one of the substances that cause blood to clot. Lupus sufferers are likely to feel tired (due to a shortage of red cells), to keep coming down with minor ailments (due to a shortage of white cells), or to bruise easily and heal slowly (due to a shortage of platelets). Taken on their own, these symptoms may not convince someone they need to see their doctor. They only become significant when part of a larger picture.

A laboratory test called a complete blood count (CBC) is needed to reveal that significance. One or another of these blood problems affects nearly all lupus patients at some time, though they are not necessarily the first symptoms the patient notices.

▶ ▶ ▶

The symptoms described up to now, some of which people may ignore or put down to the normal ups and downs of life, are the same as the ones the doctor uses to make a diagnosis of systemic lupus erythematosus. Unlike a patient, however, who is limited to his or her own subjective observations, doctors have more sophisticated ways of confirming or excluding various diseases. We will look at these tests when we return to the subject of diagnosis in Chapter 3.

> *Please note:* All the symptoms of lupus listed in this chapter, with the possible exception of hair loss following discoid lesions, clear up with treatment and leave no damage.
>
> Neither lupus, nor any other form of arthritis, is contagious, and having one kind does not predispose you to developing another.

Chapter 2

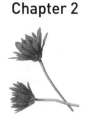

Who Develops Lupus, Where, and Why?

Estimates of noncontagious, nonreportable disease prevalence rely on some sort of official records such as hospital discharge logs, emergency-room visits, and reasons noted for school absences. It is thus possible to estimate number of heart attacks, broken legs and children suffering from severe asthma, for example, with reasonable accuracy.

Sheldon Paul Blau, M.D.
(see details of his book in Further Reading)

These days we like for numbers to be attached to illnesses. The science of who gets what, and where and when they get it, is called *epidemiology*. It is not a very exact science. So how do we get these numbers? If a disease is notifiable (see below), accurate statistics on its *incidence* (number of new cases) can be assembled. A "notifiable" disease is one that must be reported to the authorities whenever a doctor treats it. In many countries this rule applies to serious or infectious diseases, such as tuberculosis, that have public-health consequences. Likewise, if a disease is fatal or puts a patient in the hospital, it gets recorded as a cause of death or hospitalization, and as a result there may be a record of who has succumbed to it. These sorts of records are known as mortality and morbidity (illness) data. Lupus is not notifiable, and only rarely is it fatal, so we learn little about it from these records. The reason it was rated potentially fatal in the past was because only serious and fatal cases were recorded. The large number of people who had lupus but didn't die of it, or didn't even see a doctor about it, was unknown—like the body of a vast iceberg with only the fatal cases visible above the waterline.

Prevalence and Incidence

In ordinary English we use these words almost interchangeably. In statistics they measure two slightly different things. *Prevalence* usually refers to the estimated population of people suffering from a disease at any given time. Incidence refers to the number of new cases diagnosed each year. A short-lived disease like flu has a high annual incidence but low prevalence; people get it one after another but then get better. A lifelong disease like diabetes has a low annual incidence but high prevalence; only a few people develop it each year, but once they have it they have it for good. Since lupus is chronic, a person suffering from a new attack may show up more than once in the incidence statistics, but when in remission, they will not appear in the prevalence figures.

Most experts believe that there are still many invisible, uncounted cases of lupus, particularly in underdeveloped countries where there are few doctors and more serious diseases to worry about. Consequently, estimates of the number of cases and of the percentage of the population that develops lupus are constantly being revised upward. The statistics that have been gathered are mostly from developed countries with good health services and a network of medical laboratories and research organizations dedicated to the study of diseases and their treatment. In these countries scientists are funded to do population studies to ascertain who suffers from diseases, and statistics for the rest of the world are often extrapolations (scaled-up estimates) based on available data. However, where lupus is concerned not all populations or geographic localities have the same experience.

Lupus Occurs Unevenly

In the total world population it has been calculated that between forty and fifty people out of every thousand will have lupus at some time in their lives. These estimates have nearly tripled in the last forty years. This is probably not because the disease is actually on the increase, but rather because sophisticated immunological tests introduced in recent years, combined with improved diagnostic criteria, have led to mild cases of the disease being recorded. The estimates have been increased to allow for these cases.

In North America, South America, and Europe, where statistics are the most detailed, the record of new cases (incidence) ranges from 2 to 8 per 1,000 each year. A study in Great Britain has calculated that up to 20,000 people may have lupus. Estimates in the United States range from 275,000 (from a study researching women only) to a massive 1.7 million. This last figure comes from a survey commissioned by the Lupus Foundation of America and reported in 1994. It was obtained by calling people on the telephone and asking them if they had ever been told they have lupus. The researchers admit that estimating prevalence "by unsubstantiated claim" yields a figure higher than previously expected. They write, "Self-reporting studies are notoriously inaccurate as the criteria for the disease are not verified, indicating that the numbers derived from this study may not be true." Not counting this extreme estimate, it is likely that the majority of available prevalence statistics conceal a lupus "iceberg," with many more having the illness than get counted. However, national and global prevalence figures conceal massive differences in distribution between the sexes; between age, racial, and socioeconomic groups; and, to some extent, according to where people live.

Gender

Ninety percent of people who get lupus are women. Some estimates put this number even higher. It is predominantly a disease that strikes women of childbearing years (see "Age," below). This combination of characteristics suggests that vulnerability to lupus may be related to the reproductive hormone *estrogen*. Men also get lupus, as do children and women beyond reproductive age, but in every age group or other grouping, women always outnumber men. In children, in whom hormonal effects are presumably minimal, for each male, three girls get lupus. In adults, the ratio ranges from ten to fifteen women for each man. In older people (women beyond menopause, when the production of reproductive hormones is reduced) the ratio is approximately eight women for every man.

Age

As I have said, lupus strikes mostly women during their reproductive years. Sixty-five percent of patients first experience symptoms between the ages of sixteen and fifty-five. Of the remaining cases, 20 percent are affected between ages twelve and sixteen—by which age most women are sexually mature—and 15 percent after age fifty-five. Lupus does strike the very young and very old, but not sufficiently to make a statistical contribution.

Race and Geography

Different racial groups are more or less susceptible. This phenomenon is probably and principally related to the genetic differences between peoples. Tiny parts of the human *genome*—the information handed down from parent to child that programs the growth and development of the body—vary from person to person, and some genetic differences are more common in some races than others, making certain races more or less prone to certain diseases.

In every continent, there are more cases of lupus among people of African, Hispanic, and Asian descent than among Caucasians. In France, immigrants from Spain, Portugal, North Africa, and Italy are more susceptible than native Frenchmen and -women. In New Zealand, both the prevalence and mortality of lupus are higher among Polynesians than Caucasians. The vulnerability of immigrant communities may be compounded by a general tendency for lupus to be more common in urban than rural communities.

This tendency to affect immigrant communities disproportionately is something lupus shares with rheumatoid arthritis. Africans living in Africa appear less susceptible than people of African descent who live elsewhere, and certainly there is a general tendency for lupus to be more common among immigrants than among the same racial groups in their homelands, and in immigrants who move to cooler rather than tropical climes. Some researchers have suggested that this could be because immigration nearly always involves a move to cooler climes from hotter ones, and that the reduction in the amount of sunlight could play a part (see Chapter 3).

Ethnic Variables

In the 1990s the National Institution of Arthritis and Musculoskeletal and Skin Diseases (NIAMS), the agency in the United States concerned with rheumatic disorders, started recruiting several hundred lupus patients from various groups who were between the ages of twenty and fifty. Recruits were asked to take part in a study of all aspects of the disease, from clinical characteristics to psychological factors to genetics, including the contribution of ethnic origin to the incidence of the disease. The study, called LUMINA (which stands for LUpus in MInorities: NAture Versus Nurture), is ongoing as of this writing.

Is It Serious, Doctor?

Differences in the disease's severity and long-term outcome also occur between different groups. For example, black or dark-skinned people—people originating in tropical countries—have a poorer prognosis. Some studies also suggest that lupus is worse among those with less education and those from lower socioeconomic groups, though this may reflect the fact that such groups often have poorer access to health care or may fail to follow treatment and health guidelines (known to doctors as poor *compliance*).

But these days, can lupus be fatal? The short answer is very rarely. A 1955 survey showed a five-year survival rate of only 50 percent, but we now know that the study dealt with a very small, seriously ill, largely untreated group of people with the disease. With today's broader picture, it is possible to say with some confidence that lupus is only rarely fatal. Survival rates are measured over five, ten, and twenty years from diagnosis. In the mid-1990s, survival at five and ten years was close to 95 percent, and even after twenty years it was over 85 percent. If you have lupus now, with all the improvements in treatment that are available, it is highly unlikely to be life-threatening.

Lupus in Young Children

Lupus is rare in children under twelve, the age around when girls usually start their periods. Below the age of five it is exceedingly rare, although specialist physicians see a small number of cases between that age and adolescence.

Very occasionally, newborn babies develop a lupus-like rash in the first weeks of life. This is not true lupus and only occurs because the mother has lupus and some of the antibodies that cause the disease have crossed the placenta from her blood into the baby's. As the maternal antibodies die down, the rash also subsides. This condition is known as *neonatal* (newborn) lupus and is discussed in more detail in Chapter 10.

Most authorities claim that there is essentially no difference between how lupus affects young children and how it affects adults. Children who have lupus constitute a small group, so significant statistics are difficult to gather. However, some recent studies suggest that their symptoms may often be more severe than adults'. A study from the European Working Party on Systemic Lupus Erythematosus found that the pattern of symptoms in young children—and also in old people and men—differed from the pattern most typical in women sufferers. Children were less likely to have *rheumatoid factor* (an antibody that is a frequent marker of inflammation in arthritis) in their bloodstream but more likely to suffer from the butterfly rash (also known as the *malar rash*), kidney problems, pericarditis, and liver and blood complications. The rash or kidney problems were also the symptoms most likely to bring child lupus patients to the attention of a doctor.

Lupus in Men vs. Women

There are small differences in how lupus affects men compared with women. Men tend to be diagnosed at a later age, and the mortality rate one year after diagnosis (infinitesimally low in the treated population) is slightly higher. The study from the European Working Party on Systemic Lupus Erythematosus found that men were less likely to suffer from arthritis and photosensitivity than women, and that pleurisy and pericarditis were more frequently their presenting symptoms (the ones that made them consult a doctor).

Lupus in Older People

In the context of lupus, "older" is rather broadly interpreted by the statisticians as over age fifty-five—the age by which most women have passed menopause. Including men, some 15 percent of lupus cases do not appear until this age. The European Working Party on Systemic Lupus Erythematosus found that at this age new patients were less likely to present with the butterfly rash, arthritis, or kidney problems than children or younger adults. These symptoms continued to feature less (about half as often) during the course of the illness, as did photosensitivity and thrombosis. However, sufferers of late-onset lupus were twice as likely to suffer from dry eyes and mouth (*sicca syndrome*). Other studies found that the discoid rash— hard, raised plaques that sometimes leave scarring—was more common in patients who developed lupus late in their lives.

In developed countries, of course, older people are the ones most likely to be taking medication for conditions other than lupus. This introduces a group of people who, independent of age and sex, develop lupus as a consequence of taking certain drugs, a variation known as "drug-induced lupus." These are probably the only cases where the cause is emphatically certain and the cure obvious. The drug causing the problem must be stopped or changed. Drug-induced lupus is considered in more detail in Chapter 9.

Lupus in History

The name "lupus" for a skin disease has been around for more than seven centuries.

Thirteenth century. The Italian physician Rogerius describes a disease characterized by lesions and calls it "lupus." In medieval Latin the word for "wolf"—*lupus*—was also used to mean "ulcerated," perhaps because sores or ulcers that eat into the face look rather like a wolf bite.

Seventeenth century. Philosopher/physicians Paracelsus and Sennert provide clear descriptions of "lupus" skin lesions.

1828. French dermatologist Laurent-Théodore Biett identifies three types of lupus and coins the term "lupus erythemadoides" for the distinctive butterfly rash. His teachings are published by his pupil Pierre Cazenave in *Practical Summary of Skin Diseases.*

1873. Moritz Kaposi, professor of dermatology at the medical school at the University of Vienna, Austria, publishes a series of articles on lupus erythematosus, noting that patients with the rash also have other symptoms—in other words, that it is systemic. He writes, "Lupus erythematosus ... may be attended by altogether more severe pathological changes ... and even dangerous constitutional symptoms may be intimately associated with the process in question, and that death may result from conditions which must be considered to arise from the local malady."

1890. Thomas Payne, a physician at St. Thomas' Hospital, London, is the first to recognize that antimalarial drugs, long used to treat fever, may have more general healing powers for symptoms like joint pain and fatigue in lupus.

1895–1903. In a series of papers, the celebrated U.S. physician William Osler describes other organs involved in lupus—heart, kidneys, and other "mucous surfaces"—and defines the condition as both systemic and chronic (relapsing and remitting).

1941. On the basis of numerous postmortem studies of damaged organs in lupus patients, Paul Klemperer, at the Mt. Sinai Hospital, New York, proposes that lupus is a "collagen vascular" disease. This term remains in use for fifty years or more.

1948. The diagnosis of lupus moves into a new phase: Malcolm Hargraves, of the Mayo Clinic, in Rochester, Minnesota, identifies an odd-looking white blood cell, first in the bone marrow, then in the blood of people with acute lupus. It becomes known as the LE (lupus erythematosus) cell. As a result, the first blood test for lupus is devised and the number of people diagnosed rises steadily.

1954–1972. Several other anomalies are detected in the blood of people with lupus. Chief among these is an antibody that works specifically against the body's own DNA (deoxyribonucleic acid—the genetic raw material of living systems). A test for this antinuclear antibody—ANA—replaces the LE as the gold standard for detecting lupus, and lupus becomes located firmly in the family of autoimmune diseases. (Details of these sophisticated diagnostic tests are included in Chapter 4.)

1983. A group led by Graham Hughes, at St. Thomas' Hospital, identifies the antibody associated with the artery and vein thrombosis, strokes, and miscarriages that had made pregnancy so risky for lupus sufferers. The condition for which this antibody is the culprit is renamed Hughes' syndrome. (In the United States, it is more commonly known as antiphospholipid syndrome, or APS.) Treatment to counteract the effect of the antiphospholipid antibody is devised (more about this in Chapter 10).

Chapter 3

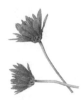

The Causes of Lupus

While no one knows what causes lupus, promising clues are scattered all over the place, like wolf prints outside a lair. Almost certainly there is no single cause, though we are able to rule out some causes.

- It is not transmitted by any infectious agent such as a bacterium, virus, or parasite. That means you can't "catch" lupus from another person, though infection may play some part in triggering it (more on this later).

- It is not caused by any known environmental agent such as industrial chemicals, toxic fumes, inhaled fibers (e.g., asbestos), microwaves, or radio towers—though, again, some environmental agent may play a part in triggering the disease or triggering a flare-up.

- It is not caused by a deficiency of any substance needed during crucial stages of embryo or infant development (e.g., vitamin, essential mineral, vital nutrient, hormone, or enzyme).

- It does not represent an allergic reaction or sensitivity to anything the patient (or the patient's mother) has eaten or come in contact with—though, again, such factors may play a part in why some people develop lupus, and lupus sufferers are as likely to have allergies as anyone else.

▶ It is not caused by a gene, or genes, handed down from parent to child. This does not mean that there is nothing in lupus sufferers' genetic inheritance that makes them more vulnerable to the disease.

Does it matter if we are unsure what causes lupus? Yes. You can treat an illness by using a mixture of experiment and observation, as ancient herbalists and witch doctors knew, but you cannot hope to cure, let alone prevent, it unless you can understand its underlying causes. As knowledge grows of what goes wrong in lupus—invariably a complex chain reaction involving more than a single bodily process—doctors have more opportunities to intervene, that is, to cut it off at the pass and ultimately stop it in its tracks.

So researchers are looking not for a single cause but for a combination of factors that lead to a person's developing lupus.

A Genetic Predisposition?

Although lupus is not caused by a defective gene handed down from parent to child, there is certainly evidence that some genetic factor is at work. When lupus is diagnosed it is not uncommon to find that the patient has relatives who have had lupus, or at the very least have had lupus-like symptoms. What seems likely is that some genetic vulnerability to developing the disease is inherited. A child with lupus in the family may be born a lupus "sleeper," with the vulnerability gene lying dormant until sparked into action by some trigger in the outside world.

Ginny's Story

While Ginny was in her mid-twenties, her husband, Bob, was posted to East Africa with the Air Force. She went with him. She had always been an outdoor person, and in Nairobi she was able to swim and ride and spend from dawn to dusk in the open. When she first noticed the rash on her face she thought she had gotten slightly sunburned, though she tanned easily and had never before been bothered by too much sun. She wore a hat and slathered on sunscreen, and the rash seemed to clear up. Then the aches and pains in her hands started. She didn't have the energy or inclination to go riding or to the swimming pool. The medical officer at the air force base murmured something about "arthritis" and suggested aspirin. Ginny suffered silently indoors. In her weekly phone call to her mother she complained of her painful hands. Her mom said, "I think you could have lupus." Ginny's aunt had nearly died during her first pregnancy, she said, and had been diagnosed as having lupus. "Come to think of it, you used to complain of pains in your hands and wrists after playing tennis when you were at school," said her mother. "We just put it down to growing pains."

Remember the mention of growing pains. The topic crops up again in Chapter 4. Experienced rheumatologists have commented on how often growing pains are mentioned in the history of people who are diagnosed with lupus as adults.

Will My Baby Get It?

When a woman develops lupus she learns that she may have problems with pregnancy. After asking "Is it all right to have children?" she will almost certainly ask, "Will my baby get lupus?" While there is a slightly increased chance of this—about 5 percent—at least the baby of a lupus mother is unlikely to develop lupus unnoticed. As explained, lupus belongs to the autoimmune family of diseases, and there is a great deal of overlap in how the immune system malfunctions and the symptoms that result from such diseases. Support for the idea that there is some inherited predisposition to developing autoimmune disease comes from several sources. First, the relatives of those with autoimmune conditions are more likely to have the same or a similar condition. About 20 percent of lupus sufferers have first-degree relatives—parents, children, or siblings—who have either lupus or some other autoimmune condition like insulin-dependent (type 1) diabetes or rheumatoid arthritis. What's more, if the blood of a lupus sufferer's healthy close relatives is tested, an additional 20 percent are found to carry immunological oddities characteristic of people with lupus, although at the time they show no outward signs of disease. These relatives may be the "sleepers" who have inherited a susceptibility gene that has so far not been triggered and become active.

Twin Studies

Comparing identical twins is the ideal way to quantify the genetic contribution to the development of a condition. Identical twins are made of identical genetic material: they share the same DNA, the basic building blocks that program living systems. If twins share a characteristic, like blue eyes or a musical ear, they are said to be *concordant*. If they differ they are said to be *dis*cordant. Identical twins start out with a high level of concordance just because they are formed from the same egg and the same DNA. If they are brought up together they also share the same environment, increasing their concordance. Fraternal twins do not come from the same egg; they are only as alike as two siblings, although born at the same time. But they will share their environment if brought up together.

Twin Studies: The Latest

In 2003, to increase our understanding of the role of genetic inheritance in developing autoimmune diseases, the National Institute of Environmental Health Sciences launched a search for same-sex siblings—twins or close-in-age brother or sister pairs—where one sibling had an autoimmune disease but the other did not. (Selecting same-sex, close-in-age pairs eliminates the variability conferred by age and sex differences.) Organizers of the study plan to enroll four hundred pairs, even though it may take a while to recruit such a select grouping. Their hope is that this research will give clearer answers regarding the role of genes that predispose susceptible individuals to whatever triggers autoimmune diseases.

The likelihood that fraternal twins will be concordant for lupus is no more than it is for siblings born at different times—a mere 2 to

5 percent. But identical twins have a much higher concordance; various studies estimate it to be from 24 percent to as high as 57 percent. From the point of view of quantifying the genetic component in developing lupus, the interesting thing is why it is no more than 57 percent. These children share not only genes; they share environment during childhood. What happened differently to the one who developed lupus? A gene for susceptibility may have been inherited, but it is clearly not the whole story.

Vulnerable Markers

Before we leave the topic of genetic connection there is another inherited component that appears to affect who succumbs to the bite of the wolf and who escapes.

About thirty years ago, when the first organ transplants took place, medical interest became focused upon why and how transplants from a donor were rejected by the recipient's body. How did each individual body distinguish between "self" and "foreign" and fight the foreign invader as vigorously and efficiently as if it had been merely a splinter or a small cut? Researchers discovered that every human cell carries an inherited code that controls a number of immune responses, including the acceptance or rejection of transplanted tissue and organs.

Everyone belongs to one or another *major histocompatibility complex (histos* is the Greek word for "tissue"), or MHC, just as all of us belong to one of several blood groups that determine what type of donor blood is acceptable for transfusion. If a recipient is in the same MHC as the donor, then the transplant will not be perceived as foreign by the immune system and has a better chance of being accepted by the body. Scientists can now pick up markers for people's MHC from their blood, just as they are able to read their blood type. These markers are called *antigens*, because they generate "anti" behavior against an invader, whether it be germs or transplanted tissue. The MHC markers also identify people who may be susceptible to certain diseases.

In the early 1970s an MHC marker was identified in 80 percent of those with the condition dauntingly named *ankylosing spondylitis,* a disabling form of spinal arthritis that strikes mostly men and had been observed to run in families. The marker was found in only 10 percent of people without the disease. Since then, MHC markers linked to several other diseases have been found, including rheumatoid arthritis, insulin-dependent (type 1) diabetes, and, yes, lupus. All these are autoimmune conditions, so perhaps it is not surprising that shared inherited factors that affect the operation of the immune system should be common to so many people with these diseases.

Since you inherit your MHC from your parents and grandparents, the same groups tend to run in families. That is why brothers, sisters, or even more distant relatives are sought whenever someone needs a transplant of bone marrow. By the same reasoning, certain MHCs will be more common in some ethnic groups than in others, which goes some way toward explaining why certain racial groups or nationalities may have a higher incidence of some diseases.

Markers for MHCs are not the only clues to understanding lupus that can be detected from tests of the patient's blood; see Chapter 4 for more on this topic.

"Sometimes It's Hard to Be a Woman"

Since nine times as many women as men get lupus, surely it seems obvious that femaleness must be to blame, right? Women have two X chromosomes and men have one X and one Y. Could there be something on that second X chromosome that makes women more vulnerable to lupus than men? Or could something on the male Y chromosome be protecting them? This is exactly how a genetic disease like *hemophilia* (a bleeding disorder) works; it is carried on one X chromosome but in the presence of a second X lies dormant. That means women carry the disease but never exhibit it. However, if a man inherits the defective X chromosome, his Y chromosome doesn't suppress the illness. He bleeds.

We know that it doesn't work like this for lupus or the differences between the sexes would be much more dramatic and the concordance of twins would be absolute.

So if not chromosomes, what about hormones? Aren't they part of what makes men and women different? We know that most women develop the disease during their reproductive years, when the sex hormones are most active. One major hospital study of all the children and teenagers who developed lupus over a period of ten years found that a substantial spurt of new cases occurred at the ages of eleven and twelve, the age of puberty.

But if female hormones were responsible for this dramatic phenomenon, you would expect the balance of hormones in those who develop lupus to be noticeably different from the balance in those who do not. (It is the balance between hormones that counts rather than absolute hormone levels.) In one study, female hormones (*estrogens*) were found to aggravate the symptoms of laboratory mice with a lupus-like illness, and male hormones (*androgens*) appeared to protect the mice. However, making an existing illness worse or better is not the same as causing it, and something that protects or cures mice might not work for humans.

Studies of assorted male and female hormone levels in humans with lupus are mostly inconclusive. Sometimes they are higher than average, sometimes lower, but not consistently so. An additional problem is that normal men and women both carry the same hormones; it is the *balance* between them that distinguishes the sexes. A significantly lower-than-average level of one hormone *was* found in both men and women with lupus. This was a form of androgen called *dehydroepiandrosterone (DHEA)*, which is a precursor of both the male hormone testosterone and the female hormones estradiol and progesterone. (The fluctuating balance of these two regulates fertility in women.) If something is in short supply, it is always possible that raising it will produce an improvement or confer protection, as it did for the lab mice, so the role of DHEA in lupus is one avenue that is being investigated. Abnormal levels of another hormone, prolactin—which in women plays a major role in enabling the production of breast milk—is being investigated in both men and women. See Chapter 11 for a discussion of drugs that affect these hormones.

It's Not What You've Got, It's What You Do with It That Counts

Before we finish with hormones as a possible cause of lupus susceptibility, let us look at what happens to them in the body. Perhaps it is not the levels, or even the balance, of hormones that makes lupus sufferers different; perhaps it is how their bodies *metabolize* hormones—break them down and put them to use. Several other conditions are caused by a failure to metabolize something useful rather than a shortage of the raw material itself. For example, type 2 diabetes is caused not by underproduction of insulin, like type 1 is, but by the failure of the body to utilize the hormone. Other diseases are caused by the inability to break down and absorb the foods that contain essential nutrients even when the diet itself is not deficient. After menopause, reduced levels of estrogens in the body make it more difficult for women to absorb calcium, even if they maintain a diet rich in the mineral, and this increases the risk of *osteoporosis*— brittle, easily broken bones (see Chapter 7).

Some studies have indeed found that lupus patients of both sexes metabolized estrogens differently from other people. This is an avenue researchers are continuing to explore.

Environmental Triggers and the Infection Connection

Why, then, does one identical twin develop lupus while the other doesn't, given that both share the same genetic vulnerability and MHC? The prevailing idea is that something in the environment triggers the disease, but since both twins are susceptible it figures that only one can have been exposed to the crucial trigger.

The most popular candidate for an environmental trigger is infection early in life. This theory is proposed for a number of diseases where the autoimmune system starts attacking the body's own tissues. The hypothesis is that, faced with an infection, the immune system gets to work to fight it, but for some reason when the infection is vanquished, instead of withdrawing, the immune system turns its guns on healthy tissue. This could be what happens in insulin-dependent diabetes, in leukemia, and in rheumatoid arthritis; some quite-unnoticed infection flips the switch and starts the antibodies off in the wrong direction.

The infectious agents that best fit the profile of a lupus trigger are viruses. Viruses are cellular parasites. There are many varieties, and what they all have in common is that they break into a living cell, hijack its reproductive system to make little virus offspring, and lurk, concealed in the body, sometimes for years. Because they hide inside cells it makes it very difficult for the immune system to access and destroy them. Nevertheless the body usually manages to generate antibodies against a virus. The presence of such antibodies in the blood of a patient therefore becomes like the footprint of where a virus has been, even when the symptoms of an acute attack have gone.

Researchers hot on the trail of a lupus trigger have looked for antibodies that might reveal that particular viruses have been there. Researchers connected with two studies, one in France and the other in the United States, thought they detected antibodies to a retrovirus, but were unable to link it to any known human variety such as HIV. Other researchers have looked for signs that infection by one of the *herpesviruses* might be responsible for triggering lupus or other autoimmune diseases. Herpes, as explained in the box titled "Know Your Virus" (on the next page), stays dormant in the body once it has invaded, flaring up occasionally—rather like lupus—usually when the body is under stress.

The evidence from these studies is encouraging; some patients with lupus, and related autoimmune disorders, did indeed appear to have elevated levels of antibodies for some of the viruses considered. But then again, these are pretty common viruses; many people have been exposed to them, so nothing very solid has been proved against them yet. Still, experts are confident they are looking in the right place for a lupus trigger in targeting viruses. Lupus expert Sheldon Blau says, "It is likely when the primary cause of lupus is found—and it *will* be found eventually—it will turn out to be a virus, whether a retrovirus, a herpesvirus or some other type that behaves in an unusual manner (or is permitted to behave in an unusual manner in some individuals, perhaps those with particular genetic characteristics)."

Blau advances yet another interesting hypothesis. Could autoimmune illnesses like lupus be triggered in people with the genetic susceptibility because they are subject to attack from *two or more* directions at the same time? In his book *Living with Lupus* (see Resources) he writes, "Perhaps the massive autoreactive activity in

---

Know Your Virus

There are many groups and subdivisions of viruses. Viruses are composed of an inner core of genetic material—the bit that reproduces itself—surrounded by a coat of protein. In diagrams they look a bit like a chestnut or a sea mine, with a spiky outer layer. The genetic core may be made of either DNA (the same material humans are made of) or a slight variation called ribonucleic acid (RNA).

The DNA group includes a large family of viruses responsible for many childhood infections of the nose, throat, and eye. The bad members of this clan are the poxvirus, which is responsible for smallpox, the milder cowpox (from which smallpox vaccines are made), and the notorious herpesviruses. The name "herpes" comes from the Latin and Greek for "creep"; it is also the root word for "reptile" or "serpent." Various members of the herpes tribe cause cold sores, genital sores, chickenpox, and shingles—conditions in which the blisters or lesions "creep" round the body. Once they have you, you have them for life. Herpesviruses are being investigated as candidates for a lupus trigger.

The RNA family of viruses also includes troublesome relatives. The members of one group, called myxoviruses, make themselves at home in the mucous lining of the nose and throat (*myxa* is Greek for "mucous"). Influenza is a myxovirus. Their close relatives, the paramyxoviruses, include measles, mumps, and scarlet fever. There is also a parainfluenza virus that causes coughs and colds. (The Greek prefix

these conditions stems from a frenzied immune-system effort to stave off simultaneous acute infections by, say, a retrovirus *and* a herpesvirus."

The Wolf's Domestic Cousins: Pets

Viruses are not the only suspects in the search for an environmental lupus trigger. A particular group of people that we haven't mentioned so far is more prone to lupus and other autoimmune disorders: pet owners.

By and large, diseases do not jump species. There are some infamous exceptions, however, like swine flu and the recent cases of new-variant CJD contracted from diseased cattle; and children often catch the fungal infection ringworm from their pets.

---

para means "beside" or "closely related to.")

Another group worth remembering is the retroviruses, a group you will hear a lot about. For some time it had been known that retroviruses caused illness in animals. Then in 1981 a retrovirus was found to be the cause of a rare form of human leukemia that damaged a group of cells that are part of the immune system, the *T lymphocytes.* This retrovirus was christened "human T-cell lymphotropic virus," or HTLV for short. Later, a similar retrovirus was identified (HTLV-2) and still later a third (HTLV-3). This last became perhaps the most famous and feared retrovirus in history. It is now better known as the human immunodeficiency virus—HIV. Over a period of years it wreaks such havoc in the immune system that, left untreated, it leads to death from AIDS.

But back to lymphocytes. In addition to T lymphocytes—the ones implicated in the rare leukemia and in HIV—there are also B lymphocytes. When a foreign invader is detected, B lymphocytes produce antibodies specifically to attack that particular invader (the antibodies are antigen-specific). Two types of T lymphocytes work alongside these B cells. T "helper" cells do exactly what the name implies; they support the work of B cells, partly by cleaning up the debris of the battle against foreign invaders. T "suppressor" cells do just the opposite. They act like a damper or governor, making sure B cells don't get overenthusiastic in their activity. The T suppressor cells fail to do their job in several autoimmune diseases.

The wolf's domestic cousin, the pet dog, is implicated in lupus. The fact that dogs develop lupus became widely known in the U.S. when, in the early 1990s, the first President George Bush and his wife, Barbara, both developed a condition called Graves' disease, an autoimmune illness of the thyroid gland. At the same time it was discovered that the Bushes' dog, Millie, had lupus.

Tess's Story

Tess, a university student, developed lupus while taking finals. Her family had been watching anxiously for the illness ever since Tess had started her periods, because her mother also had lupus. She had discovered the illness during the 1950s, when she had become pregnant and then lost the baby. Tess managed to complete her finals, and once she started taking an antimalarial drug the rash that had appeared on her face, back, arms, and chest began to calm down. During summer vacation she took it easy, and it looked as though the first flare-up was behind her. Then she noticed a funny thing. Her cat Jinxy was off her food, was reluctant to move from her cushion, and when she did move she appeared stiff and in pain. Chunks of her fur even started to come out. Tess took Jinxy to the vet, who discovered that the cat had severe ulcers in her mouth. He called the condition "stomatitis," a general term for inflammatory disorders of the mouth. But Tess was convinced her cat had lupus. "Cats don't get lupus," insisted the vet, but he agreed to give Jinxy a corticosteroid injection. Within a few days she appeared to get better.

Unusual anecdotes do not constitute proof. However, where dogs are concerned there is solid evidence that they do suffer from a form of lupus, exhibiting symptoms similar to humans, including arthritis, skin lesions (mostly around the nose) that are aggravated by sunlight, and kidney problems. The canine condition also shows a similar pattern of flare-up and remission, and responsiveness to the same drugs. So could there be transmission between pet and owner? A small study published in *The Lancet* in 1992 offers some support to this notion. A group of dogs owned by patients with lupus was compared with an outwardly healthy group owned by non-sufferers, and also with a group of dogs diagnosed as already having lupus. To all outward appearances the lupus patients' dogs were perfectly healthy, but when their blood was tested it was found to have significantly higher levels of the antibodies characteristic of lupus sufferers' blood than were found in both the healthy control animals and the dogs known to have lupus! Something linked the lupus humans and their dogs, but what exactly? A link between pet ownership and a higher incidence of other autoimmune diseases has also been found, though it is not always supported by blood tests demonstrating that pets and owners carry the same antibodies.

Scientists are always reminding us that just because two things happen at the same time, or follow each other, it doesn't mean that one *causes* the other. It could be coincidence. It could be that both events share a common cause, some environmental trigger or infectious agent that affects pets and humans who live together. One thing is certain, however: Pets and their human owners don't share the same genetic susceptibility!

Other Possible Environmental Triggers

One or two other possible lupus triggers have been investigated.

Smoking is known to trigger a flare-up in people with lupus. A number of recent studies point to smokers being as much as two times more susceptible to lupus as nonsmokers. A similar effect has been noted with other autoimmune diseases.

Evidence that an environmental pollutant is contributing to an illness is usually found in the form of *clusters*—that is, an increased incidence of a disease in particular localities or geographical areas. Clusters of juvenile leukemia were discovered in areas around a nuclear power plant in Sellafield, England, suggesting that the plant was in some way triggering the illness. Pesticides and certain industrial toxins have been implicated in other diseases. Lupus clusters are very rare. One was reported in Arizona in the mid-1990s, and exposure to pesticides or other industrial contaminants was postulated as a possible cause but not backed up by firm evidence.

A number of therapeutic drugs are also known to cause lupus or, more correctly, lupus-like symptoms. It's not true lupus because once the drugs are withdrawn the condition disappears and does not recur (more about drug-induced lupus appears in Chapter 9).

▶ ▶ ▶

This has been a long chapter because, given the uncertainty surrounding the disease, it has been necessary to consider many factors in order to explore its possible causes. When the various steps that lead to lupus are eventually understood, a much shorter chapter will be required—though longer chapters may then have to be written on treating, curing, or even preventing lupus!

Chapter 4

Diagnosing Lupus, Part 1: In the Doctor's Office

For patients, the experience of lupus starts with symptoms: how they feel and what they see—rash, aches and pains, hair on the comb, fatigue. The doctor is also first presented with the patient's symptoms. Some can be seen, others discovered by asking questions (taking a history), and yet others detected through the doctor's knowledge of how the healthy body works and what signs indicate things are going wrong.

Unless faced with the classic butterfly rash, few general practitioners are likely to diagnose lupus in the office. Even with painstaking history-taking and examination (the first two parts of diagnosis), certainty may evade them. The fact that fatigue, depression, or general aches and pains are frequently the first presenting symptoms of many conditions can easily throw the primary-care physician off the trail of lupus. Furthermore, although a battery of laboratory tests have now revolutionized the diagnosis of lupus, a doctor needs to know which tests to order.

Lupus patients often see several doctors before they are correctly diagnosed. In 2002 the American Autoimmune Related Diseases Association reported that the majority of those with serious autoimmune diseases had experienced difficulty obtaining a diagnosis. Many had been told their symptoms were "in their heads" or that they were suffering from stress. No fewer than 45 percent had been told they were hypochondriacs! A wise physician may order some of the basic tests as soon as he or she has seen the patient, but will also refer the person to a rheumatologist.

Taking a History

History-taking involves the person detailing her symptoms to the doctor, and the doctor asking questions to gain maximum information. The aim is to narrow down the possible explanations—disease candidates—and then to eliminate them and arrive at a differential diagnosis. Suppose the patient has fatigue, fever, rash, hair loss, or aches and pains; the doctor needs to rule out infection, allergic reaction, or a hormonal imbalance, to name just a few conditions that might cause similar symptoms. Suppose the doctor advances to the conclusion that the patient has some autoimmune condition, or even one of the connective tissue diseases. He or she is still only at first base. How can the field be reduced to one?

To make this task easier, the American College of Rheumatology (ACR) publishes a list of diagnostic criteria for each of the connective tissue disorders. These are basically checklists of symptoms and signs that have been found in international studies to accompany confirmed diagnosis of each condition. They are not a substitute for the individual doctor's examination of the individual patient, but they do provide guidelines for what should be covered in an examination, and they ensure that the exam is as thorough as possible. ACR's diagnostic criteria for lupus were first drawn up thirty years ago and have been revised several times. The important physical symptoms are those listed in Chapter 1. Some are more significant than others because they are highly specific to lupus (see the box "Specificity and Sensitivity," on page 40). Taken together they build a composite picture of the illness.

Symptoms Detected in the Doctor's Office

Here is a list of physical symptoms of lupus as classified by the ACR:

▶ *Butterfly (malar) rash*—This is the oft-cited classic symptom, "probably more due to its picturesque name than its prevalence," says Sheldon Blau. The rash may not be itchy or painful, but may burn slightly on exposure to sunlight. It usually disappears, leaving no mark.

▶ *Discoid lesions*—These are circular, raised, red, scaly plaques. More common in men and in late-onset (older) lupus patients, they were once considered a separate form of the disease because they are often the only lupus symptom patients have. These lesions can leave scarring and permanent hair loss when they heal.

▶ *Photosensitivity of the skin*—This rash specifically follows exposure to sunlight or fluorescent light. Although it occurs in no more than a third of lupus patients it is often a presenting symptom and is highly specific to lupus, particularly if it is accompanied by lupus-type symptoms in other parts of the body.

▶ *Ulcerative sores*—These blister-like sores are sometimes, but not always, painless. They affect the mucous lining of the mouth and throat, and occasionally the vagina. If they're painless, a dentist may notice them before the patient does.

▶ *Arthritis*—The other classic symptom of lupus, arthritis causes pain during motion, as well as stiffness, tenderness, and swelling of peripheral joints (hands, arms, feet, and legs). It is caused by inflammation. Three-quarters of lupus patients present with it, and 90 percent suffer from it at some time, but although common, this symptom is by no means specific to lupus. Literally hundreds of conditions cause joint pain; it is at the top of the list of symptoms seen by primary-care physicians. At first, lupus-related arthritis is indistinguishable from rheumatoid arthritis. Subsequent laboratory tests separate one cause from another.

Sensitivity and Specificity

Laboratory tests supplement the physician's know-how and intuition, but they are still far from perfect. And they are imperfect in two ways that also apply to clinical signs. First, they identify some but not all who have a disease—that is, they sometimes give a false negative result. Second, they give a positive result for some people without the disease—a false positive. If the test picks out, say, ninety-nine out of every hundred people with the disease, it is said to be extremely sensitive. If it only gives one false positive result for every hundred people *without* the disease, it is said to be extremely specific.

So does it matter? Surely 99 percent accuracy is pretty good? Think of it like this: You are a guard with an X-ray gun that enables you to see if anyone coming through a checkpoint is carrying a hidden bomb. If the test for a hidden bomb is positive you blow the terrorist to kingdom come. If the X-ray gun sees nothing, the traveler is an innocent tourist whom you let pass with a wave. Now suppose your X-ray gun shows a shadow that looks just like a hidden bomb. You blow it up and—oops, it was a harmless tourist carrying a video camera! Or suppose your X-ray gun misses a terrorist with a bomb and he gets through undetected. Just as bad.

So it is with false negatives and false positives for disease. It is not too serious with a disease like lupus, but suppose you get a false negative for HIV? That person may go on to spread the life-threatening disease, unaware of being at risk. And if you give someone a false positive for HIV a life will be damaged even though that person may not have the disease. This is why medical scientists rely on the sensitivity and specificity of tests so much, and it is unusual for them to base a diagnosis on just one test. As with clinical signs, wherever possible several different tests are relied upon, and if results are negative the tests may be repeated, just in case they were false.

▶ *Chest/heart problems*—The most common of these is pleurisy: inflammation of the membrane enclosing the lungs. But patients may also develop pericarditis: inflammation of the membrane surrounding the heart. The patient usually complains of chest pain especially when breathing deeply. Like arthritis this is not a symptom in any way specific to lupus, and a physician will first wish to exclude acute causes like infection or cancer. Again, laboratory tests help sort one cause from another.

▶ *Kidney disorder*—The kidneys are sometimes known as the "silent" organs in lupus because inflamed kidneys produce no obvious symptoms for patient or doctor. (Pain around the kidneys is more likely to be caused by something completely different, for example a urinary-tract infection or a kidney stone.) The clearest evidence that the kidneys are in trouble is fragments of protein or blood cells leaking into the urine that make it look cloudy. Healthy kidneys filter out protein and blood, leaving the urine clear and sterile. Another sign that the kidneys may be inflamed is raised blood pressure. Testing blood pressure and urine is a standard part of a thorough medical examination, so physicians will usually pick up any kidney involvement. About half of all lupus patients may have a degree of kidney involvement at some time; reports vary. Once again, taken alone, kidney problems are not specific to lupus.

▶ *Signs of neurological disorder*—Lupus affects blood vessels all over the body. Inflammation of those in the brain may cause headaches, severe migraines with flashing lights, nausea, or vomiting, or even alarming symptoms like seizures or signs of mental disturbance, for example exaggerated and irrational fears (phobias) or hallucinations. These brain symptoms have only recently been recognized as indicative of lupus; in the past some lupus sufferers were diagnosed as having schizophrenia. But the accumulation of symptoms in other parts of the body confirms their underlying inflammatory origins.

Diagnosis: Craft or Science?

Diagnosis, doctors are taught, is like Gaul: divided into three parts. You take a history from the patient; you examine; you do tests. You then collate and compare this information with the features of diseases known to you in the hope of making a match or at the very least a differential diagnosis. "It can't be this, this, or this; so, by elimination, it must be that." In practice, doctors hardly ever work like this.

Doctors are fond of joking to each other that they can diagnose their patients "at the office door." And of course, much of what family doctors see is the same—coughs, colds, stress, general fatigue, and old age—but the saying also prevails because they become practiced in reading their patients' ills from subtle signs. In the words of one doctor, "The eye of the experienced beholder is worth a laboratory-load of tests." This diagnosis by intuition or divination conjures up the old idea of doctor as magical medicine man, though in practice it is actually diagnosis by expertise gained through experience. The *Oxford Handbook of Clinical Medicine* (OHCM) calls this practice "diagnosis by recognition," and it probably applies less to lupus than to other conditions; nevertheless, it is interesting to consider this and the other styles of diagnosis.

Diagnosis by recognition. This is the "office door" diagnosis that comes with years of experience. It impresses both patient and medical student (when a student happens to be present). It is hard to quantify, harder still to teach, and it is not infallible. The OHCM says 20 percent of such diagnoses are demonstrably wrong. Fortunately, the modern laboratory detects such error.

Diagnosis by reasoning. This is the Sherlock Holmes technique. The evidence for and against each candidate disease is considered, with the aim of excluding it. Whatever remains after elimination is the diagnosis, however unlikely. This system fails because the list of candidates may not include the actual illness in the first place, or because the reasons for dismissing some candidates are faulty. This is why it belongs, like Holmes, in fiction, says OHCM.

Diagnosis by "Wait on Events" (WoE). This was a popular diagnostic technique in the distant past when there was little doctors could do to treat or cure a condition. Inaction was in many cases less harmful than action that might turn out to be wrong. A celebrated doctor observed that, of the patients who came to his consulting room, 50 percent would get better whatever he did, 25 percent would get worse whatever he did, and 25 percent might actually benefit from what he could do. The advantage of WoE was that he reduced the people needing help by the half who recovered, and his success rate doubled to 50 percent of the remainder. Of course it's not as simple as that, but WoE still often figures in a modern doctor's notes. Even in chronic conditions like lupus, a pattern, or an additional confirmatory symptom, may appear while you are waiting for those all-important laboratory tests.

Diagnosis by hypothesis. This is the classic scientist's approach, not unlike Sherlock Holmes'. Postulate a diagnosis and then try to disprove it. It's thorough, but lengthy, so in some ways not unlike WoE. Something will probably happen to the patient that illuminates things while the doctor is hypothesizing.

Diagnosis by computer. This increasingly popular technique is as new as WoE is old. It has its advantages: The computer gives access to a range of expertise in addition to the doctor's own. It may throw up some curious options—the computer can't see the patient coming through the surgery door—but among them may be something the doctor hadn't thought of.

▶ ▶ ▶

Faced with a long row of check marks in a list of the clinical signs for lupus, a primary-care physician would treat the presenting symptoms but also refer the patient to a rheumatologist. He or she would also order laboratory tests that would help confirm his or her provisional diagnosis of lupus. These tests are explored in the next chapter.

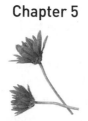

Chapter 5

Diagnosing Lupus, Part 2: In the Laboratory

Around a hundred and fifty years ago, observed or "clinical" symptoms, as described in the last chapter, were all the doctor had to go on to diagnose lupus (or any other illness), and they were not usually conclusive. These days, doctors can call up a raft of sophisticated laboratory tests. A sample of blood or of another bodily fluid or tissue may be taken in the doctor's office, but the analysis is completed by machines and skilled technicians in the pathology laboratory. Advanced and expensive imaging technology that reveals details inaccessible to the human eye is also available. It makes you realize why primary-care physicians often complain that they are just a staging post in modern medicine.

The American College of Rheumatology (ACR) diagnostic criteria include important evidence that can't be detected at a primary-care consultation but requires laboratory tests. Up to this point it has been sufficient for us to say that most lupus symptoms are caused by inflammation—inflammation prompted by an unexplained malfunction of the immune system. But if we are to go further and explain how the disease is detected in the laboratory, we need to look at the inflammatory process and its causes in more detail.

Inflammation: The Good News and the Bad

Inflammation feels the same wherever it occurs, whether in the form of a sore throat, a splinter, a corn, or arthritic joints. It causes warmth, redness, swelling, and pain. The amount of inflammation, hence the severity of the symptoms, is usually proportional to the severity of the injury or infection.

The body is a self-maintaining, self-repairing organism. Inflammation, though it may feel unpleasant, is actually a signal that the attack/defend/repair armory of the immune system is at work. There are a number of weapons in this armory—WMD: weapons of microscopic destruction, if you wish—each of which has a slightly different role to play in coordinating attack and in returning the immune system to normal afterward. White cells, or lymphocytes (the name indicates cells produced in the lymph glands, among other places), are the foot soldiers of inflammation. As mentioned earlier, they are subdivided into B cells and T cells. The T cells have their own role in fighting viruses and tumors, and they also influence the behavior of B cells.

At the start of an attack, B cells produce antibodies specifically tailored to repel the invader. "Helper" T cells assist in this task, along with back-up troops called *complement*. These proteins complement the activity of antibodies in neutralizing the antigen. The embattled cluster of warring antigen, antibody, and complement is called an *immune complex*. If you think of it like the line of scrimmage in a football game, or a knot of big guys in a barroom brawl, you can see why inflammation causes so much damage to surrounding tissues, particularly the kidneys in lupus: What results is the equivalent of broken glass, splintered furniture, and torn curtains. The objective is to destroy the antigen, but a lot more gets damaged in the process. During the battle, damaged cells at the site of infection or injury send out alarm calls in the form of chemical messengers called *cytokines* to summon the foot soldiers. Many different forms of these chemical messengers are active in inflammation: Some put out the call to battle; others tell the troops to back off when the enemy is vanquished. T "suppressor" cells come onto the scene later to tell the B cells to back off when their work is done (more on them later).

While the inflammation rages, the blood supply to the battle-field is increased, producing redness and warmth, and the body's temperature rises. Clear fluid and white cells pass through the walls of the blood vessels into the surrounding tissues, causing swelling and pain as a result of the pressure upon the tissues. The fluid di-lutes poisons and is mildly antiseptic, and the white cells engulf, break down, and remove any foreign particles, such as bacteria, that they encounter, cleaning up the battlefield so that reconstruction can begin. The fluid—called inflammatory exudate—has the same capacity as blood to clot, and it will seal off clean wounds, such as those resulting from a surgical operation or minor infection. The clot causes the edges of the wound to stick together so that new tis-sue can grow to heal the breach.

If the enemy is not swiftly routed, pus may form, composed of inflammatory exudate and broken-down cells of dead bacteria and white cells. (You may need to blow your nose, clear your throat, or lance an abscess.) The bone marrow and other blood-forming tis-sues are stimulated to produce yet more white cells. Ultimately, in the normal course of events, inflammation is self-limiting: T sup-pressors call a halt once the infection is cleared or the wound healed. However, in autoimmune diseases like lupus and rheuma-toid arthritis, "it ain't necessarily so."

Immune System Malfunction

Autoimmune diseases affect players in the immune system. For ex-ample, the AIDS virus attacks T helper cells, depleting them so that people with the disease eventually succumb to a range of op-portunistic infections that a healthy immune system would nor-mally take in its stride. In lupus, as in rheumatoid arthritis, the problem is an overactive immune system. The antibody-producing B cells increase eight- to tenfold, and the T suppressor cells, de-signed to suppress antibody production once the alien invader has been vanquished, are in short supply. B cells that produce antibodies with no obvious enemy to attack are called *autoreactive*—in other words, reacting to the body itself—and one of the things they appear to attack is immature T suppressor cells, which may explain the shortage of mature active ones in people with lupus.

A healthy immune system, like other body systems, depends on balance—on the right number of actors playing their parts at the right time, delivering the right lines, and then leaving the stage. For more than thirty years scientists have known that in lupus, B cells continue to produce antibodies when there is nothing to attack, and they have been trying to fathom why. Is it that the B cells are still getting messages (via those important cytokines) to attack, or are they failing to get the message (from other important cytokines) to stop? And is that because too many "Attack!" messages go out, or too few "Back off!" messages? Is the problem too many or too few message senders—helper T cells or suppressor T cells—or is it that the right messages get scrambled and don't get through to the overactive B cells? When you realize how complex the interaction of these immune-system actors is, you can see how difficult it is to unravel which part of the play has gone wrong. From the point of view of scientists trying to put things right, it means lots of different places where they can try to intervene.

There is a colorful cartoon version of the inflammation battleground, plus a depiction of what goes wrong in lupus, on the Lupus Society of Alberta website (see Resources).

Messages in Blood

From the point of view of the doctors trying to make a diagnosis, there are lots of potentially malfunctioning components to look for in the lupus patient's blood. The blood is the body's transport system, and a great deal of information can be obtained by unpacking the things carried around the body in the bloodstream at any one time. Other bodily functions are also informative: urine, the fluid inside joints or spinal cord, blood-pressure readings, and recordings of the electrical activity of the heart and brain. But in lupus blood tests are vital. So if you have it, resign yourself to having a lot of needles stuck into you.

In addition to the clinical symptoms outlined in the last chapter, the remainder of the ACR diagnostic criteria for lupus are detected from blood tests. Here is a list of them:

▶ *Hematological (blood) abnormalities*—These usually show up in a complete blood count (CBC), a procedure as basic as taking a pulse or blood-pressure measurement. Almost all lupus patients will have some abnormal factor in their blood at some time in their illness. There could be a shortage of *erythrocytes* (Greek for "red cells"), the red blood cells that carry oxygen around the body. Shortage of red blood cells is called anemia (the names for things in blood often end in *-emia,* from the Greek for "blood"). Or there may be a shortage of white cells, the ones that fight disease, a condition called leucopenia (Greek for "white" and "deficit"). Or there could be a shortage of blood-clotting cells, called *platelets* or *thrombocytes* (Greek for "clotting cells"); this leads to excessive bleeding, in the form of either bruises or the bursting of small blood vessels in the skin, or sometimes it leads to the failure of a wound to heal properly.

Doctors also test the rate at which red cells in unclotted blood form sediment at the bottom of a test tube, a simple, nonspecific test called the *erythrocyte sedimentation rate (ESR).* If there is inflammation or increased autoimmune activity in the body, the cells break down and the sediment collects more rapidly. The test is simple but rather crude, with several limitations. For instance, sedimentation may speed up for all sorts of reasons, for example because the patient has an infection or from any number of inflammatory conditions other than lupus; and indeed patients can be quite ill but have a normal ESR. Then again, it slows down if the patient is taking certain common drugs, like penicillin, diuretics, or vitamin A. But a doctor who has taken a thorough history will be alerted to this complication.

Blood may also be tested for C-reactive protein (CRP), which is produced by the liver in response to inflammation. Like ESR the presence of CRP is an indicator of acute inflammation, though not specifically for lupus. It is more sensitive than ESR because it is only rarely found to be abnormally high in the blood of healthy people. Both ESR and CRP are useful when it comes to monitoring the success or otherwise of treatment.

▶ *Immunological disruption*—As explained, in lupus there is a massive increase in the number of antibodies circulating in the patient's blood. Several different sorts are found, and four are highly significant for lupus:

1. The antiphospholipid antibody, which is responsible for an illness called *antiphospholipid antibody syndrome* or APS (a syndrome is a group of symptoms that occur together). Another name for the condition is "sticky" blood syndrome or Hughes' syndrome, after Graham Hughes, head of the Lupus Research Clinic at St. Thomas' Hospital, in London, and one of the foremost experts on the disease (see his books or Triona Holden's *Positive Options for Antiphospholipid Syndrome (APS)*, in "Further Reading"). In 1983, Dr. Hughes' team described a disorder characterized by blood clotting in both arteries and veins. Pregnant patients with the problem had a tendency toward recurrent miscarriage, and all sufferers were at higher risk for stroke. (A stroke occurs when a clot of blood that has formed in a blood vessel breaks loose and travels to the brain, causing loss of function and sometimes death.) APS affects perhaps 1 to 2 percent of the

general population, but a very high proportion of lupus patients, to the extent that its presence is highly suggestive, if not conclusive, of the disease. The discovery was also important because it showed that not all the features of lupus were caused by inflammation. (More about APS antibodies appears in Chapter 10.)

2. About 40 to 50 percent of lupus patients have an antibody known as anti-Sm (the "Sm" has no medical meaning; it comes from the name of the patient in whom it was first identified). The test for it is not particularly sensitive (a high percentage of people with lupus do not test positively), but it may be unique to lupus, hence highly specific (no false positives).

3. Elevated levels of anti-DNA, an antibody to the basic building block of life (deoxyribonucleic acid, found in the nucleus of all human cells), occur at some stage in at least 50 percent of people with lupus. Some researchers believe it may be unique to lupus, making it highly specific, though not particularly sensitive (many lupus sufferers test negatively).

4. Finally, there is an antibody found at high levels in the blood of people with lupus that, although not exclusive to them, is considered so significant that it warrants the status of an ACR diagnostic criterion. *Antinuclear antibodies* (ANA) appear to react indiscriminately against material released from the nucleus of a cell when it has been destroyed. Although patients with other diseases—rheumatoid arthritis, liver disease, and some infections—as well as those on some drugs, also react positively to this test, a very high proportion of lupus patients (in some studies between 90 and 100 percent) test positive, which makes it one of the most sensitive tests available, although

again, not highly specific. Yet another sign that an abnormal degree of cell destruction has taken place (all
that broken furniture) is the presence of unusually
high levels of freely circulating DNA in the blood of
lupus patients. DNA properly belongs *inside* the nucleus of a whole cell, not wandering about in the
bloodstream.

The last two antibodies listed are noteworthy and distinctive.
They are not the kind present in the blood because the patient had
been exposed to and has fought off an infection like tuberculosis.
Nor are they the kind stimulated deliberately by vaccination to protect people against a future attack of an illness like measles. These
are antibodies characteristic of autoimmune conditions; they do
battle with the body's own cells. These antibodies don't react to in-
tact tissues and organs, but rather to broken-down pieces of cells released during the autoreactive battle.

With few exceptions, normal cells in the body die eventually;
the body is in a continual process of renewing and replacing itself,
disposing of old, worn-out cells and building new ones, all with no
disruption to the smooth running of the body as a whole. The
process of normal, programmed cell death is known as *apoptosis*,
from two Greek words that mean "falling away." One avenue that
scientists are exploring is that in autoimmune diseases something
goes wrong with normal apoptosis. Instead of quietly falling away,
"elderly" cells totter on in a decrepit state, continuing to promote
inflammation and abnormal autoreactive activity (see Chapter 11).

Other Signs, Other Diagnostic Techniques

I know this has been a long, rather difficult chapter, and it isn't over
yet. Please hang in there and read this section, even if you have
skipped reading about some of the complicated antibody tests.

Some symptoms that aid diagnosis used to be on the ACR list
but have been dropped. One is hair loss. About a quarter of lupus

patients experience hair loss, but there can be alternative explanations. Another is a condition known as *Raynaud's phenomenon,* which is a bit like frostbite and can exist independently of, as well as in association with, lupus. Raynaud's phenomenon is caused by a spasm of small blood vessels—*vasospasm*—which shuts off the circulation to the extremities, usually the fingers but occasionally the ears, nose, or toes, so that they turn white, then blue with cold, and then red and painful. More about this condition can be found in Chapter 9.

Other significant changes may show up in the blood of lupus patients; for example, the amount of complement—the antibody-support troops who figured in the description of inflammation earlier in this chapter—may be depleted as a result of prolonged inflammation. Other, more interesting, though not specific, antibodies may also add support to a diagnosis. But for now that's quite enough about antibodies.

The St. Thomas' Criteria

Before we can move on from diagnosis to the important business of how lupus patients are treated, I would like to return for a moment to the concept that says, "the eye of the experienced beholder is worth a laboratory-load of tests" that we encountered in Chapter 4. Graham Hughes, who heads the lupus unit at St. Thomas' Hospital and who was responsible for identifying Hughes' syndrome, says in his book *Lupus: The Facts* that the ACR list, although invaluable for the purpose of *classifying* lupus, is restrictive when it comes to diagnosis. "It narrows the scope for lateral thinking in clinical medicine, something which lupus, above all, allows us in abundance," he says. Dr. Hughes has drawn up an alternative diagnostic list of fourteen lupus symptoms (eleven of which are summarized below) that may be detected in the doctor's office from observation or the patient's history. They have, he admits, no statistical justification. They are based "solely on the experiences gained in a huge clinical practice." (He also lists additional evidence that may be noted in laboratory tests, but these three criteria are not included below.)

▶ *"Growing pains."* In the U.K. and the U.S. this is a label widely used for joint pains occurring during childhood and teenage years. While usually considered benign, they are often severe enough for the child to be taken to a doctor. Some patients give a history of "rheumatic fever," a label that persists, at least in the U.K., despite the condition's almost total disappearance.

▶ *Teenage migraine.* This symptom is associated with antiphospholipid (Hughes') syndrome. Many patients over age thirty with cerebrovascular accidents (blood clots that migrate to the brain) give a past history of recurrent spontaneous abortions (miscarriages) in their twenties and "migraine headaches" in their teens.

▶ *Infectious mononucleosis.* Prolonged periods of patients having missed school due to infectious mononucleosis (sometimes called "glandular fever") is a recurrent theme among lupus sufferers.

▶ *Severe reaction to insect bites.* In Dr. Hughes' book *Lupus: The Facts,* he says, "The skin is a major organ affected by lupus. It would be surprising if hypersensitivity to insect bites were not an important phenomenon in lupus."

▶ *Recurrent miscarriages.* Dr. Hughes again: "To be precise, this criterion is not truly a lupus criterion, but is an indicator of those lupus patients with the antiphospholipid or Hughes' syndrome. Indeed, in our lupus pregnancy clinic we believe that if APS patients are excluded, then lupus itself is not a cause of recurrent spontaneous abortion."

▶ *Allergy to Bactrim or Septra (a common antibiotic drug) or sulfonamide (an old sulfur-based antibacterial drug; also called sulfa drug).* It is quite common for patients to report not only a history of severe rashes and other adverse reactions to Septra, but also that the clinical onset of lupus coincided with their taking of the drug.

▶ *Agoraphobia (fear of open spaces) or claustrophobia (fear of enclosed spaces).* It is known that the central nervous system is involved in lupus. Dr. Hughes believes that evidence of abnormal fears in a patient's history indicate a pre-lupus warning. He says, "The history, varying from panic attacks in shops to fear of motorway [highway] driving, for example, is sometimes protracted, lasting months or years. In many cases, the history is not volunteered, or the episodes are considered unrelated or 'something from the past.'"

▶ *Finger flexor tendonitis (difficulty in extending the fingers flat caused by joint and tendon inflammation).* The patient says, "I cannot say my prayers." Dr. Hughes values this as a lupus pointer because it varies from the pattern of finger-joint inflammation seen in other connective tissue diseases like rheumatoid arthritis.

▶ *Premenstrual exacerbations (problems).* All rheumatic diseases are influenced by the menstrual cycle, and none more so than lupus. Some patients are almost immobilized during the two to three days preceding menstruation. Dr. Hughes: "It is my practice in some cases to alter the dose of medication during this time. Although difficult to quantify, I believe that significant premenstrual disease flare is sufficiently prominent in lupus to be included in this alternative list."

▶ *Family history of autoimmune disease.* This is self-evident common sense. Dr. Hughes comments, "In old-fashioned history-taking, the family history is important. Lupus is genetically determined, and the presence of other autoimmune diseases in the family (including thyroid disease) is worthy of inclusion in the clinical scoring system."

▶ *Dry Schirmer's test (the doctor sticks a sliver of blotting paper into the lower eyelid)*. According to Dr. Hughes, the test is "highly irritant and only if the patient has some abnormality of the tear duct—as in lupus or *Sjögren's syndrome*—will the paper remain dry. In a patient with vague or nonspecific symptoms, a bone-dry Schirmer's test points towards one of the autoimmune diseases."

In conclusion, Dr. Hughes says, "All of us can diagnose lupus in the presence of a butterfly rash, *nephritis* [kidney disease], and alopecia [hair loss]. The challenge comes at the other end of the spectrum; the atypical case; the mild case; the differential between real disease versus no organic disease whatsoever; the ailing teenage daughter of a known lupus patient."

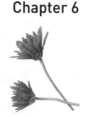

Chapter 6

Treating Lupus with Drugs, Part 1

Lupus is a fiendish beast to track down, hence the immense effort to arrive at a diagnosis. Once the doctors are pretty sure they have it in their sights, however, the plan of attack can be made. Lupus has many manifestations, and treatment is inevitably tailored to the severity of the patient's symptoms. The protocol for treating the illness comprises four main drug groups:

1. Painkilling nonsteroidal anti-inflammatory drugs (NSAIDs)

2. Antimalarials

3. Steroids

4. Immunosuppressants

Up to the middle of the last century, lupus was so poorly understood that doctors had little science to guide them; hence they adopted the "let's-see-if-this-will-do-any-good" principle still somewhat in use today. Serendipity and the law of averages mean that such pragmatism quite often produces a hit. There may also be disasters, and success via serendipity does not greatly advance our understanding of the disease process. The other snag of the approach is that even when a drug appears to work against some symptom of a disease, unanticipated and harmful side effects, or the emergence of subgroups of people who are particularly vulnerable to them, emerge only later. These are some of the reasons why *therapeutics*— that is, treatment of illness with drugs—advances these days by means of properly controlled trials that demonstrate effectiveness and side effects before new, experimental treatments are licensed for general use (see the box "Randomized Clinical Trials (RCT): The Therapeutic Gold Standard," on pages 58–59).

The Problem of Polypharmacy (Taking a Lot of Drugs at Once)

Before looking at the drugs used to treat the various symptoms associated with lupus, here's a word about taking drugs in general. "Polypharmacy" means "many drugs," and it refers to problems arising from the unwanted duplication of medications or from adverse interactions between drugs. Most of us get used to taking acetaminophen for a headache, a course of antibiotics for a bladder infection, or an antihistamine for hay fever, but these common medications are all taken in response to recognized symptoms, taken alone, and stopped once the symptoms subside (or once the course is complete, in the case of antibiotics). The drugs prescribed for lupus are less symptom-specific. In addition, lupus patients have the same common ailments requiring medication as the rest of the population, so at times they may find themselves with a veritable pharmacy laid out on the dressing table. What's more, the fatigue and emotional ups and downs that often accompany lupus can play havoc with memory and attention, potentially causing problems with a patient's drug regimen.

The advice of the experts is as follows: Write your medication schedule down—which pill, how many, at what time of day, and whether it is to be taken before or after food. Ideally, check each one off the written list as you take it. You should probably also make a note of any drug that doesn't agree with you. Some drugs can increase photosensitivity, for example, already a problem for many with lupus; others produce side effects such as an upset stomach or rashes in some people. If you experience side effects from any drug, make sure to record which one and exactly how it affects you, and make sure it is listed as problematic on your medical and dental records.

The problem of polypharmacy is not unique to people with lupus. The preventive regimens designed to protect against heart disease and other conditions of old age—for example, menopausal symptoms, high blood pressure, raised cholesterol, and diabetes—

Randomized Clinical Trials (RCT): The Therapeutic Gold Standard

The idea of using the scientific method to test the effectiveness of drugs or other medical procedures is a relatively modern concept. Curing people has historically been as much about faith and luck as it has about medical understanding or effective treatment. But as the causes and mechanisms of disease emerged from mystery and superstition, so the physician's ability predictably to alter the course of disease—to intervene—increased.

The first example of what is now regarded as the gold standard for clinical trials—the randomized, controlled trial, or to give it its high-carat denomination, the randomized, placebo-controlled, double-blind trial—took place just after the Second World War in 1948 when Austin Bradford Hill set up a trial of streptomycin, an antibiotic derived from soil fungi discovered a few years previously, to measure its effectiveness in tuberculosis. Patients with advanced pulmonary (lung) tuberculosis (TB) were randomly assigned to one of two treatment groups. If doctors are allowed to choose which patients receive a new active drug and which are allocated to the control group, there is always the risk that they will put the patients with the best prognosis into the active group, thus skewing the outcome. When, in addition to patients being randomly assigned to either the treated or control group, patients don't know whether they are on the active drug or not, the trial is known as "blind." If, in addition, the medical team looking after the patient and running the study is not told which patient is in which group, the study is "double-blind"; neither the patient nor the medical staff know who is in which group. This prevents any hidden psychological bias for or against the new treatment. Clinical studies usually

mean that many of us take a lot of pills starting in middle age. Lupus patients are old hands at it long before that.

Charlotte's Story

Early in the summer of 1976, Charlotte, a senior in high school, was outdoors studying for final exams. She developed a fiery rash and felt generally unwell, but somehow she managed to keep going and waited to visit the doctor until summer vacation started. At once he recognized the classic butterfly rash, organized a battery of tests, and told Charlotte she had lupus. The symptoms subsided over the summer with little medication.

---

measure the effect of a new treatment against a *comparator:* either the standard treatment of the day—it would be unethical to withhold all treatment from a sick person for research purposes—or, in nonfatal conditions, unlike TB, against a nonactive dummy pill (a placebo) to conceal from them whether they are taking the active treatments or not. Patients with some illnesses—depression, for example—may show marked improvement when receiving a placebo. This response to treatment, albeit with a nonactive compound, is called the placebo effect.

In the Hill study of streptomycin, 107 patients were enrolled. When the results were unblinded it was discovered that 14 of the 52 patients on standard treatment had died (remember that these were very ill people), but that only 4 of the 55 patients who had been given the active drug had died. Streptomycin really worked.

The supremacy of the RCT was reinforced in the early 1950s by trials of the Salk polio vaccine. It was tested using an elaborate double-blind trial on nearly two million children in the U.S. These early successes, together with early failures of clinical testing procedures—for example, thalidomide, an effective drug for morning sickness in early pregnancy, was found to have damaged the fetus developing in the womb—led to the establishment of laws in Europe and the United States governing the testing of experimental drugs. These days, before a drug is approved for general use it must be tested against these standards. As David Healy says in his book *The Antidepressant Era* (Harvard University Press, 1997), "Randomized, placebo-controlled, double-blind trials are the appropriate means, indeed almost the only scientific means, to establish the efficacy of a treatment."

Charlotte took a year off and went backpacking across Europe. Somewhere in what was then Yugoslavia she developed cystitis (bladder infection) and found herself trying to communicate with a local doctor in the rudimentary German they both spoke. "Keine penicillin" (no penicillin) insisted Charlotte, who knew she was allergic to the drug. Unfortunately she couldn't remember the name of the antibiotic that her family doctor did prescribe for her. She certainly didn't know the German word for lupus. The local doctor prescribed a sulfa drug, and within two days Charlotte broke out in a rash—not just on her face, but on her hands, lower arms, and ankles. Even though it was November, the drug had potentiated Charlotte's photosensitivity.

Nonsteroidal Anti-Inflammatory Drugs (NSAIDs)

The acronym NSAIDs—pronounced "en-sayeds"—is used freely in talking about dear old aspirin and its younger siblings. They are used to treat such a wide range of conditions that two important things about them are easily overlooked: They kill pain, and they reduce inflammation without belonging to the *corticosteroid* family of drugs. Corticosteroids are also powerfully anti-inflammatory and very effective in the treatment of lupus (see Chapter 7). However, they pack a payload of side effects, and they also have some rather disreputable relations: the anabolic steroids used by some athletes to enhance performance.

In the first half of the twentieth century, high doses of aspirin—the oldest member of the NSAID family—were the standard treatment for rheumatoid arthritis, juvenile arthritis, and lupus patients with arthritic symptoms. However, once the dosage and side effects of these drugs were studied in properly controlled trials it emerged that good old aspirin had quite a few serious side effects. It irritates the lining of the digestive tract, causing indigestion and intestinal bleeding, and it may also affect the liver. People with lupus, it appears, are more likely than most people to be prone to abnormal liver reactions to aspirin, especially in high doses, so the develop-

ment of NSAIDs about forty years ago was welcomed by rheumatologists and arthritis sufferers alike.

NSAIDs suppress pain by interrupting the messages sent from
the site of the pain to the brain. The cytokines—the chemical messengers that become so overexcited in rheumatic conditions—produce substances called *prostaglandins* that cause inflammation.
Aspirin and the NSAIDs work by interrupting this process. That's
why you will sometimes hear them called "prostaglandin inhibitors."
When production of prostaglandins is reduced, so are pain, swelling,
and stiffness. They are good as a first-line treatment for these symptoms because they are fast-acting (as anyone who is a fan of aspirin
knows, it offers pain relief within half an hour). Inflammation and
swelling take a little longer to be affected, but they start to go down
within a week or so on a regular course of NSAIDs.

Just as experienced users learn that one painkiller works better
for them than another, trial and error are usually required to find
which NSAID is effective and produces the fewest side effects for
individual lupus patients, because NSAIDs also have side effects.
The most common is indigestion, a result of the irritation the drug
causes to the lining of the stomach, which can ultimately lead to ulcers. More refined versions that aim to reduce inflammation without damaging the gastric lining have recently been developed and
are known as "coxibs" or "COX-2 inhibitors." (To learn how these
work and about their drawbacks, read the box "Good and Bad
COX.")

When NSAIDs are used to treat rheumatoid arthritis or lupus
they are primarily being prescribed to reduce inflammation and thus
are required in higher doses than for a headache or muscle strain.
Finding the right drug and establishing the effective dose with mini-
mum side effects may take some time. Although these are for the
most part tried and tested, garden-variety drugs, some of which are
even obtainable without a prescription, in the doses used to treat
arthritic symptoms they need close monitoring. In addition to the
risk of a wide range of side effects, some people are allergic to them.
Furthermore, they may interact with other drugs patients may be

---

Good and Bad COX

NSAIDs work by blocking an enzyme known as *cyclooxygenase* (COX), which contributes to the production of prostaglandins that in turn release platelets that promote blood clotting and protect the gut, kidneys, and blood. This is why prostaglandin-inhibiting drugs can damage the gut and kidneys, producing the common side effects of increased gastrointestinal bleeding and upset stomach. A little more than twelve years ago, scientists discovered that there were in fact two sorts of COX enzyme: COX-1, which acts to protect the gastric lining, and COX-2, which is only found in inflamed tissue and which is produced in response to stimulation by those overexcited cytokines that characterize autoimmune diseases. The race was on to inhibit COX-2—the bad guys—while leaving COX-1 to carry on the good work.

---

taking. Bottom line: Remember to always report any unusual symptom or reaction to your doctor right away. It is estimated that as many as thirty million people worldwide take NSAIDs every day to control pain and inflammation. Family doctors are familiar with their side effects.

There are currently four COX-2 inhibitors (coxibs) on the market (see the box "NSAIDs Used to Treat Lupus"), and two more are in the pipeline. At first there was much excitement about these improved NSAIDs; in clinical trials of people with arthritis they controlled pain and inflammation without as many nasty gastric side effects. However, in September 2004, follow-up research in a large number of patients revealed that there was a slightly increased risk of "cardiovascular events" (heart attack or stroke) for those on a coxib called rofecoxib or Vioxx, and the makers withdrew it.

Inevitably this raised questions about the others. The argument goes that normally, although COX-1 tends to promote thrombosis (blood clotting), it is inhibited by the action of COX-2, so that blocking COX-2 would suggest that unopposed COX-1 would indeed increase cardiovascular risk. On the other hand, inflammation is also implicated in cardiovascular events, and therefore controlling inflammation by blocking COX-2 should be protective. As

NSAIDs Used to Treat Lupus

First, think for a moment about drug names. Drug names belong to no spoken language and are almost impossible for the layperson to pronounce or remember. They are assembled piecemeal by the people who develop the drugs and are intended to provide clues as to what's in the medications or how they work. But drug names only do this for experienced pharmacologists. Just to complicate matters, each drug has at least two names: its chemical name, which describes its active ingredients, and its trade name or brand name, which, like Coca-Cola or Pepsi, is capitalized. Trade names are meant to be catchy and easier to pronounce than chemical names, but they often aren't. And they vary from country to country, which makes them even more difficult to recognize.

There is an unspoken belief among doctors that patients don't really need to know more about their drugs than is included in the patient information leaflet enclosed in the packaging (and which aptly carries the acronym PIL). They think it will make you worry. But if you know the names of your drug and can get on the Internet, you can find out a lot, both good and bad, about your medication.

Here is a list of NSAIDs commonly used to treat lupus:

▶ NSAIDs: salicylates (aspirin—acetylsalicylic acid in fancy dress; Bufferin, Ecotrin, Encaprin), ibuprofen (Advil, Motrin IB, and Nuprin), fenoprofen (Nalfon), ketoprofen (Orudis, Oruvail), piroxicam (Feldene), naproxen (Aleve), diclofenac (Cataflam, Voltaren), nabumetone (Relafen)

▶ COX-2 inhibitors: Celecoxib (Celebrex), valdecoxib (Bextra), etoricoxib (Arcoxia)

Rofecoxib (Vioxx) is the drug that has been withdrawn following the side-effect scare. Lumiracoxib (Prexige) is currently still undergoing clinical trials.

usual with this sort of medical conundrum, "further studies are called for." Meanwhile, wise old family doctors observe that not only are coxibs now tarnished with the "cardiovascular event" brush but that in practice some patients taking them still experience the gastric side effects they were supposed to avoid. *And* they cost a great deal more than aspirin or standard NSAIDs. "I foresee them disappearing from the scene," said one experienced doctor.

Treating pain is only half of treating lupus—and NSAIDs only a quarter of the drug groups doctors prescribe. For more about additional powerful drugs, turn to Chapter 7.

Chapter 7

Treating Lupus with Drugs, Part 2

Doctors are instinctively conservative. If they believe it is safe to "wait and see"—to avoid intervention and allow the body to correct itself without medical assistance—they probably will do so. If the patient's symptoms, even temporary ones, are sufficiently severe to make "wait and see" too miserable to endure, they will still first choose the mildest of treatments, the one with the least side effects. Only if matters become serious do they go in with the big guns. This is why we have discussed NSAIDs first for the treatment of lupus. Although not side-effect free, they are well known and comparatively mild. The other drugs in the lupus pharmacy have more serious potential side effects, but balancing this risk, they are generally more effective.

Antimalarial Drugs Are Antilupus

The first group of drugs found to be helpful in lupus was originally designed to attack the malaria parasite, a great example of the serendipity that occasionally blesses the "let's-see-if-this-will-have-any-effect" approach. The oldest antimalarial drug, quinine, was tried experimentally in lupus as early as the 1890s (see "Lupus in History," in Chapter 2), and related drugs were used successfully in the 1920s to heal the skin lesions associated with discoid lupus. Several quinine derivatives are still prescribed today, particularly hydroxychloroquine (Plaquenil), chloroquine (Aralen), and quinacrine (Atabrine). Of the three, hydroxychloroquine is most commonly prescribed because it has the lowest side-effect profile.

Treating malaria in its active phase involves reducing fever, so perhaps it is not surprising that antimalarials do this for lupus sufferers too. But they also help with skin lesions, joint inflammation, and fatigue. Characteristically for a serendipitous discovery, there is no clear explanation as to why they should have this effect. They are immunosuppressive. (A study done in Africa showed that antimalarials used conventionally to treat active malaria reduced the response to vaccination, when in fact a protective immune response is the desired effect.) They are also antiviral and anti-inflammatory, though via what mechanism is unclear, possibly by suppressing the production of prostaglandins (as do NSAIDs) or those chemical messengers of inflammation, the cytokines (see Chapter 5). They have two other clearly beneficial actions: They are sun-blocking—valuable to lupus sufferers who are so often hypersensitive to light—and they lower cholesterol, one of the soluble fats transported in the bloodstream that contribute to cardiovascular disease and the production of blood clots. This is good news for people with lupus, who often have clotting problems, especially during pregnancy, and good news for everyone else too.

... and Now the Bad News

There are of course side effects with antimalarials. There is a small risk of the usual upset stomach (about one patient in five), ringing in the ears (*tinnitus*), and occasionally headaches, but the major concern is damage to the retina of the eye.

When hydroxychloroquine is first prescribed it is usually given in quite high doses—up to 400 milligrams (mg) a day—and it can cause temporary visual problems: blurred vision or a "halo effect" around lights. This is reversed once the dose is reduced. Finding the optimal dose for an antimalarial is quite difficult because the drug does not become effective for at least two weeks, sometimes longer, so this initial side effect can be decisive in determining whether the drug can be used on any given patient. Graham Hughes employs a "juggling" drug regimen with antimalarials if a patient has severe skin complications. If 400 mg of hydroxychloroquine daily causes vision problems, he reduces the dose by using a different antimalarial (quinacrine) on alternating days. (Quinacrine, also known as mepacrine, is not a first-choice antimalarial because it has its own vision side effects and can also produce slight yellowing of the skin and eye whites.)

The more serious vision side effect of antimalarials was seen more frequently in the past when high doses were used with less caution. It takes the form of pigment deposits in the retina—the area at the back of the eye where images are formed and relayed to the brain. This condition is called *macular retinopathy* and if allowed to continue undetected can lead to blindness. For this reason most hospitals keep a close watch on patients who are taking the drug. They are advised to protect their eyes from strong light *of all sorts* and *at all times*, and to wear high-quality sunglasses, indoors as well as out, especially if they may be exposed to fluorescent or halogen lighting. In addition the eyes should be examined regularly by a qualified ophthalmologist. The frequency of such examinations can be as little as every few months, but not less than once a year.

If these precautions are observed there is evidence that antimalarials may be taken for months, or even years, and that in addition they may protect against lupus flare-ups.

Douglas' Story

Douglas developed lupus in middle age. At first he attributed the arthritic symptoms to wear and tear; it was only when the distinctive discoid rash appeared on his scalp that his doctor realized it was lupus. Hydroxychloroquine was prescribed, and after a few weeks the symptoms cleared up. But when the medication was stopped, the symptoms returned. Douglas went back on the antimalarial, this time for months. It was only when he had his routine eye test nearly a year later that the ophthalmic optician discovered that there was damage to the retina. Douglas had noticed nothing unusual; as far as he was concerned his sight was normal. His doctor changed the medication, very apologetic that he had not insisted on Douglas' having an ophthalmic checkup sooner. Subsequent eye exams showed that the damage was not progressing. Douglas was lucky; sometimes the sight continues to deteriorate even when the drug is stopped.

In the past, antimalarials were always discontinued during pregnancy because of the risk that they might affect the developing fetus. However, an increasing number of studies now suggest that successful pregnancies can be completed by women who are taking hydroxychloroquine, though some obstetricians still prefer to err on the side of caution.

Corticosteroids

Does the hair stand up on the back of your neck at the mention of these drugs? Once highly thought of, they have acquired a bad reputation. When the first drug—*cortisone*—was launched in the 1940s it demonstrated such dramatic reductions in inflammation that it was hailed as a wonder drug, a "cure" for rheumatoid arthritis and lupus, and earned its discoverers, Philip Hench and Edward Kendall, a Nobel Prize.

But in the wake of the rave reviews for the miracle cure came serious side effects (mostly because the drugs were being used in very high doses at the time): weight gain, increased blood pressure, easy bruising and slow healing, cataracts, muscular weakness, elevated blood sugar causing problems with diabetes, less resistance to infection because the immune system was being suppressed, and, with long-term use, thinning of the bones (osteoporosis). Corticosteroids were no longer the flavor of the month.

Corticosteroids are, in fact, laboratory versions of hormones occurring naturally in the body. Human steroids are produced mostly by the adrenal glands, but also by the testicles and ovaries. They help control *metabolism* (how the body generates energy and disposes of waste), the development of sexual characteristics, immune function, the balance of fluids in the body, and its tolerance of stress. There are many steroids with different functions; the sex hormones (testosterone, estrogen, and progesterone), adrenal cortical hormones, bile acids, sterols, anabolic agents, and oral contraceptives are all steroids. Corticosteroids are not the same as anabolic steroids, the ones taken by weight lifters to build muscle. The role of corticosteroids is protective: They maintain the fluid balance in the body and help it cope with stress; along the way they reduce inflammation.

Doses and Delivery Regimen of Steroids in Lupus Treatment

In the treatment of lupus, the role of steroids is anti-inflammatory. Nowadays the pros and cons of corticosteroids are better understood, and their use, delivery, and dosage have been refined. They have probably advanced the treatment of lupus more than any other drug, and almost every person with lupus will take them at some time or other, on a short-or a long-term basis. Doctors prescribing them follow strict guidelines.

Getting the dose right—not too much, not too little—is central to the administration of steroids. Inflammation is the healthy response to infection, so if it is suppressed (by drugs) the patient becomes vulnerable to infection; hence it is essential that the dose is kept as low as is effective. In Graham Hughes' experience, a seriously ill patient may briefly require as much as 60 mg daily, reducing to 30–40 mg after one or two weeks. Milder cases might receive 15–20 mg daily for the first few weeks, reducing to a maintenance dose of 5–10 mg a day. Reducing the daily dose of steroids must always be done gradually and with the cooperation of the patient. It is possible to reduce high doses on a steeper gradient, but a reduction of a dose that is lower than 20 mg must always be extremely gradual—as little as 1 mg a month—in Graham Hughes' experience.

(This fine-tuning can be hampered by the difficulty of finding 1 mg tablets, requiring the patient's cooperation in neatly cutting up pills with a razor blade.)

A number of steroid drug regimens may be employed. They are most commonly taken by mouth; the most widely used drug is prednisolone (or prednisone). ACTH (adrenocorticotrophic hormone) is an injectable form of steroid that is administered twice weekly, and methylprednisolone is given via a drip into a vein. This can obviously only be done in the hospital, but for seriously ill people it can be a useful way of delivering large doses of steroids with surprisingly few side effects. (When steroids are taken by mouth they are available in a coated form to reduce the usual unpleasant gastric side effects.) At the other end of the dose scale is the practice of prescribing steroids to be taken on alternating days, to allow the natural source of steroids—the body's own adrenal glands—to reboot. One of the principle side effects of steroid treatment is that the body, recognizing that large amounts of the stuff are washing around, cuts back on home production. This is why coming off steroids must be done gradually—to let the adrenal glands limber up and get back into production.

Taking low-dose steroids, for example 7.5 mg a day, even for a limited period, causes other side effects. Two are quite common: sleep disturbance and increased appetite. As has been explained, steroids control metabolism, which in turn determines when energy and attention levels go up and when they come down, and, accordingly, the cycles of attention and sleepiness that constitute your body clock. Some people who take steroids find their body clocks totally reversed; they're wide awake at three in the morning and sleepy at three in the afternoon, as though they had been working the night shift or had just returned from the other side of the globe with jet lag.

Taking high doses of steroids over long periods triggers the side effects that gave the drugs their bad name: muscle weakness, increased blood-sugar levels (sometimes full-blown diabetes), and osteoporosis. High doses are usually only given for acute emergencies in lupus, and rarely for more than a short period. (Treatment for os-teoporosis is covered later.) One of the lesser-known side effects is mood disturbance: depression or the opposite, mania. If the family has a history of psychiatric problems it should always be reported to the physician before a patient takes steroids.

Corticosteroid Drugs Used to Treat Lupus

Here is a handy list of them: prednisone, prednisolone, methylpred-nisolone (Medrol), dexamethasone, triamcinolone, betamethasone, cortisone, hydrocortisone, and adrenocorticotrophic hormone (ACTH) injections.

Immunosuppressive Drugs

Lupus is an autoimmune disease, so you might think it obvious that it should be treated with immunosuppressive drugs. In fact, im-munosuppressants were developed for a quite different medical condition. Fifty years ago, when the first successful human organ transplants took place, rejection was a great problem. The body re-ceiving the transplant recognized the organ as a foreigner and the immune system attacked it. Drugs to suppress this natural process were essential if transplanted organs were to survive. Some drugs al-ready in existence were found to have immunosuppressant action (serendipity scores again), and others have been developed since. These have been tried as treatment for conditions like rheumatoid arthritis and lupus in which an overactive immune system is part of the problem. In lupus they clamp down on the overproduction of antibody-producing B cells. They also interfere with rapidly divid-ing, proliferating (multiplying) cells, hence are also used to treat cancer. Immunosuppressants are used in much lower doses to treat autoimmune diseases than they are for organ-transplant rejection or cancer. Nevertheless they are potent drugs, and their powerful action may spread to other, healthy cells that are not their desig-nated target.

Their side effects are considerable, so they are only given if the disease becomes serious—if the kidneys are inflamed (nephritis), for example—or if milder drugs are ineffective, and always under very close medical supervision and with constant monitoring.

The two immunosuppressants used most frequently to treat lupus are azathioprine (Imuran) and cyclophosphamide (Endoxana, Cytoxan). Two others may be used as backup: methotrexate (Folex, Mexate, Rheumatrex) and cyclosporin (Neoral, Sandimmune). An additional, relatively new drug, mycophenolate mofetil, or MMF (CellCept), has distinguished itself in the support of kidney transplants and looks promising in the treatment of lupus, although it has yet to establish a long track record. Let's take a closer look at each of these.

Azathioprine

This is the immunosuppressant used most widely in the management of lupus. Although it lowers resistance to infection, it has an otherwise quite acceptable side-effect profile. It has even been used for children with lupus and sometimes for pregnant women. The dose given, usually between 100 and 150 mg a day, is based on body weight. It has been used to treat nephritis and has been continued successfully for a period of years. On the evidence of blood tests it also appears to have a beneficial effect on other aspects of lupus.

Cyclophosphamide

Studies over the past twenty years suggest that this drug is even more effective than azathioprine, especially when it comes to life-threatening kidney disease, and it is the most likely to be prescribed when heavy-duty therapy is indicated. It may be taken by mouth, like azathioprine, or by injection, often by what is known as *pulse therapy*. This involves delivering relatively high doses of the drug straight into the vein (intravenously) at specific intervals of days, weeks, or months. This drug may also be used in conjunction with an antimalarial, or with a corticosteroid such as prednisolone or methylprednisolone. This last combination has been very successful in maintaining prolonged lupus remissions.

Methotrexate and Cyclosporin

Methotrexate has revolutionized the treatment of rheumatoid arthritis because of its powerful effect upon joint inflammation. It can be helpful in lupus if arthritis is the chief problem and may also help with skin rashes, but it is not the first drug of choice for the condition. Cyclosporin, which modifies the immune system in a slightly different way from other immunosuppressants, may be helpful in some cases of lupus, but on the downside it carries serious and distinctive side effects, one of which is elevated blood pressure. Since this is a major problem in lupus patients who have kidney involvement, cyclosporin is definitely at the bottom of the list for lupus.

Mycophenolate Mofetil or MMF (CellCept)

By contrast, this addition to the immunosuppressant drug list has recently increased sharply in favor. It was initially launched, like its brothers, to treat organ rejection after transplant; the first studies to demonstrate its use in the treatment of autoimmune disease were published in 2003. It showed itself to be as effective, if not more so, than pulse therapy cyclophosphamide and with a much lower side-effect profile.

For obvious reasons new drugs are first used on the most seriously ill patients, often those who have failed to respond to standard drug therapy, on the principle of "nothing to lose." MMF was compared with cyclophosphamide for the treatment of lupus patients with severe kidney disease. The newer drug's reduced side effects gave it another leg up over the older drug: Fewer patients withdrew from treatment. All too often distressing side effects contribute to patients' deciding that they would rather go off the drug than put up with them anymore—what doctors call *noncompliance*. The most effective drug is useless if patients can't stand taking it.

It remains to be seen if MMF will prove as successful in treating patients with less severe manifestations of lupus—that is, those with less to lose by abandoning treatment.

Treating Drug Side Effects

Of course, people with lupus don't have to give up a drug to avoid side effects. Some effects can be treated with yet more drugs.

Infection

Immunosuppressants and corticosteroids reduce the body's ability to fight infection by depressing the production of white blood cells in the bone marrow. Every effort must be made to avoid exposing lupus patients who are on these drugs to infection. The herpesviruses, which cause shingles and cold sores, are a particular problem, but they can be treated with an antiviral called acyclovir. Cystitis (inflammation of the bladder), another common problem with pulsed cyclophosphamide, responds to a drug called mesna. Bacterial infections can be treated with antibiotics.

High Blood Pressure

Nothing is more important for lupus patients with kidney involvement than controlling blood pressure. To do the topic justice, it requires a book to itself. Fortunately there are now very reliable, low-side-effect treatments for elevated blood pressure. The regimen that best suits lupus patients with kidney problems is a *diuretic*—a drug that reduces the amount of water retained in the tissues—plus a *calcium antagonist*, which works on the walls of blood vessels to reduce pressure.

High Blood Cholesterol

Half the population of the United Kingdom and an estimated one-third of the population of the United States has a blood cholesterol level that puts it at risk of coronary heart disease, so most of us are aware of the value of reducing dietary fat, particularly the "bad" saturated fats (the ones in dairy products and meat). Elevated cholesterol is even more of a risk for lupus sufferers; fortunately there is a class of drug known as *statins* that support a healthy diet and may provide a range of other benefits as well. Needless to say, on no account should a person with lupus smoke. It is a major aggravation of high cholesterol, high blood pressure, and heart disease.

Osteoporosis

This loss of bone density leading to easy fracturing and poor healing is one of the most serious results of prolonged or heavy use of steroids. Most patients on long-term steroid treatment undergo regular bone-density scans and take calcium supplements and vitamin D supplements to help their body metabolize the calcium. If these prove insufficient, a drug from a group called *bisphosphonates* may be prescribed. Examples of these are alendronate (Fosamax) and risedronate (Actonel).

▶ ▶ ▶

People with lupus who also have antiphospholipid (Hughes') syndrome have a major problem with thrombosis (blood clots), and usually have to take medication to counteract this condition. Such medications are called *anticoagulants,* and they are discussed in Chapter 10.

Chapter 8

Do-It-Yourself Lupus Management

This is a book about coping with a chronic illness. We've talked about research, doctors, laboratory tests, and drugs. They are all there to inform and help you. But when you come home from the hospital or doctor's office and go through your front door, you are on your own. Day-to-day coping is up to you, hopefully with the support of friends and family.

This chapter is in some ways the most important one in the book. Yes, you need to know what lupus is all about, but above all you need the know-how, strength, and resourcefulness to grapple with the wolf in its lair. The wolf will always be with you, but you can put it on a leash and make it heel.

At first it will seem daunting. It may feel as though your life will never be the same. Persevere. Break the problems down into bite-size pieces and deal with them one by one. Each person with lupus will have different priorities. For one the fatigue will be the major obstacle, for another the painful joints. Yet another may feel devastated by the damage to self-esteem caused by the skin rashes. Or maybe it is the mood swings that get you, or the headaches, or the upset stomach. Whatever your particular bane, there is something that you, together with doctors and the right drugs, can do to overcome it. Being active in disease management is empowering; it restores your self-confidence. It doesn't mean you can't ask for help if you need it. Getting constructive advice from experts, family, friends, or colleagues is a practical coping strategy in itself.

Most of this chapter focuses on managing the unpleasant symptoms that typically accompany lupus. Let's take a look at a few of these.

"I Feel Tired All the Time"

Fatigue is probably the most common symptom of lupus and the most intractable. How can you find the energy to cope when you feel like a wet dishcloth all the time? Take comfort in the fact that medication almost always helps. Once the drugs start to take effect, things begin to feel better. Get the doctors to confirm that you are not anemic or that you don't have a lower-than-normal level of thyroid hormones or essential minerals, all of which can be corrected.

Meanwhile take stock of your life. Lupus fatigue is known by a variety of names: super-fatigue; wipe-out fatigue; a different kind of tired. Acknowledge it, and then treat it—with rest if necessary, in whatever dose is required. Jot down the situations or activities that make you feel most exhausted, and find ways of avoiding them, modifying them, or correcting the fatigue they cause.

Gillian's Story

Gillian is a financial high-flier, a specialist in private/public partnerships. When lupus struck, in her early thirties, her biggest problem was finding ways to cope with business travel. It was bad enough commuting back and forth between the city and her home in the suburbs, but crossing time zones and then immediately afterward being expected to be bright and bushy-tailed in a business meeting was impossible. "I got the company to let me work from home at least three days a week," she explains. "My laptop is networked so that I am in touch with everyone wherever I am, but I don't have to sit on the train for two hours every day to go into the office. Working from home is so much more flexible. If I need a nap, I can take it. If it's easier to work at night—the steroids sometimes do that to me—no one bothers me; they pick up my messages when they come in the following morning. As for business trips to New York, or, worse, to Tokyo, I allow an extra day so that I can sleep for at least ten hours before I have to perform. And, of course, I tend to increase my drug dose before those trying times."

Coping with fatigue, as Gillian found, requires a mixture of cessation, adaptation, and compensation. Don't drive yourself into the ground, and don't blame yourself. If you have always been a busy, industrious person it is important to tell yourself that rest is therapy, not laziness, let alone sin. Lupus fatigue should not be ignored in some mistaken stoicism or guilt trip.

"I Look Awful"

An illness that affects the skin, especially the skin of the face, is devastating because in addition to bringing discomfort it damages your self-image. You don't just feel ill—often, you know you look ill.

Fortunately, medication usually banishes a lupus rash, and there is a lot you can do yourself to make sure it stays that way. Once again it involves making note of what prompts a lupus flare *in your case*. The most likely cause is light of some sort. More than a third of people with lupus are photosensitive. As with sunburn, the fairer your skin, the more likely you are to be vulnerable. It doesn't mean you have to stay indoors, but when outside you should probably wear long sleeves, long pants, and a broad-brimmed hat, and use a high-SPF sunscreen generously and repeatedly wherever your skin is exposed. Surveys reveal that nearly everyone fails to use sufficient sunscreen, and the places most likely to be neglected are the temples, the ears, and the back and sides of the neck. (Women, or men whose workplace is tolerant, could do worse than grow long hair and bangs.) And when you choose a sunscreen make sure it is non-allergenic. People with lupus are more prone than most to allergies. Watch out for sunscreens that contain para-aminobenzoic acid (PABA) or padimate; quite a few people react badly to these substances.

You will gradually get to know your limits, but until you do, approach high-reflectivity locations such as beaches, ski slopes, and boats with extreme caution. Reflected light can make such locales as lethal in winter as they are in summer. If you are a light-sensitive lupus sufferer you may also need to be wary of some forms of artificial light. Unshielded fluorescent bulbs emit significant amounts of ultraviolet light, as do halogen lamps. One woman with lupus found that her skin was affected by repeated exposure to the "flashbulb" in the photocopier—a hitherto unsuspected occupational hazard.

Like Charlotte (see Chapter 6), you may find that your photosensitivity is aggravated by certain drugs or foods. A list of things to watch out for appears in the box on the next page, "Things Known to Increase Photosensitivity."

Allergy is another trigger for the skin symptoms of lupus, and, as explained, people with lupus are more prone than average to allergic reactions. The fact that the human body can absorb things via the skin has been successfully used by drug manufacturers to their advantage. If a drug can enter the system this way it avoids having to pass through the hostile environment of the stomach. However, the preservatives, colorants, perfumes, and other additives used in cosmetics, aftershaves, detergents, and a range of common manufactured products that come in contact with the skin in the course of modern life may prompt an allergic reaction and, in a lupus sufferer, a flare-up. Nail polish contains the same sulfonamides that sparked Charlotte's lupus; a whole range of cosmetic substances, including permanent hair colorings, have been known to set off allergies—again, especially among people with lupus.

This doesn't mean that from now on you must go naked and unadorned. Nothing would be more likely to make you feel miserable about your appearance. It does mean that you should adopt an attitude of extreme caution and constant vigilance about what goes on your skin. In the kitchen and during housecleaning, rubber gloves are de rigueur; those delicate, reverse-handed gloves used by doctors won't make you clumsy. And when you go shopping for cosmetics look for the hypoallergenic selections.

Things Known to Increase Photosensitivity

Some foods that derive from plants that contain chemicals called psoralens may aggravate photosensitivity. The most prominent are lemons, limes, celery, parsnips, parsley, and figs. Even people without lupus have been known to suffer nasty skin reactions if they have spilled fruit juice on their skin on a sunny day.

Drugs that have this effect are many. The ones that people with lupus are most likely to encounter are antibiotics (not just sulfa drugs, but also tetracyclines), an NSAID called piroxicam, a diuretic (water pill) called hydrochlorothiazide, some blood-pressure medications, antidepressants, and antiseizure medications. Photosensitivity is always mentioned among the side effects listed in the patient information leaflet (PIL) of a prescription drug. For a detailed list of medications with this potential side effect, go to the website www.emedicine.com/derm/topic108.htm (see Resources).

If you do have a flare-up of your lupus rash, the accessibility of the skin as a route for medication works to your advantage. Steroid skin creams reduce the itchiness of both malar and discoid rashes (1 percent hydrocortisone creams are available over the counter), and the side effects common with oral corticosteroids are rare with topical products. Calamine lotion is also helpful for itching, as are warm baths with colloidal oatmeal or a bath-oil rub. Some people find glycerine soap less drying than the regular kind. Sicca syndrome, also known as Sjögren's syndrome (see Chapter 9) after the physician who first described it, contributes to overall skin dryness. Ask your doctor to recommend an unperfumed pharmaceutical moisturizer, as opposed to a cosmetic product, that you can use regularly all over your body.

If self-help remedies fail you, there are two new immunosuppressive topical treatments that the doctor can prescribe for you: tacrolimus (Protopic) and pimecrolimus (Elidel). Launched in 2002, these creams are not steroids and so far appear to have minimal side effects.

"Sometimes I'm So Depressed I Want to Die"

Being ill makes anyone feel fed up. The realizations that you are ill and it hurts, that it's mucking up your life, and that it could go on for the rest of your life can feel like a prison sentence.

In fact, people with lupus are not depressed solely as a reaction to having the illness. The disease itself can cause problems in the brain that lead to depression. People diagnosed with lupus often have a history of depression, and the good news is that it lifts once they are treated. The bad news is that some treatments—steroids, for example—can in themselves cause mood disruption. Disease and treatment don't affect everyone in the same way. If you do continue to feel disabling depression once your lupus is treated, your doctors may suggest antidepressant drugs, at least while you come to terms with things.

However, you can also do some things to help your body cope with your feelings.

Exercise

One of the most effective ways of lifting mood is with regular, consistent exercise (although exercise may also be used symptomatically, to relieve stress or improve mood). Since exercise is also a helpful way to maximize movement and range in arthritic joints and an even better way to stave off the risk of osteoporosis, it comes highly recommended for people with lupus. Some people also find that it helps with fatigue, and exercise is, of course, to be recommended for everyone who values a healthy lifestyle.

It's a well-known fact that exercise gives you a natural high. Some people become addicted to it, work out to achieve it, and feel down if they can't get their regular fix of it. The explanation is thought to be that exercise releases natural body chemicals called *endorphins*, which appear to reduce pain and generally to lift the spirits. Exercise also concentrates the mind because it involves effort. Unpleasant, intrusive thoughts recede. Your mind and body become focused on the present. Those who don't exercise are skep-tical of these claims. Get into an exercise routine and discover the truth.

Exercise doesn't necessarily have to mean lifting weights or go-ing to the gym, though the use of moderate weights—around 2½ pounds—can, among other benefits, be helpful in warding off os-teoporosis. Brisk walking, swimming, dancing, and golf (if you're walking rather than riding in the cart) all keep the joints and mus-cles active, encourage deep breathing, and pleasantly occupy the mind. If your joints are swollen you will need to strike a balance be-tween rest and gentle exercise. If in doubt consult your doctor or a physiotherapist.

Maintain Meaningful Contact with Others

Which "others" only you know. Keep doing things with your chil-dren, keep going to church or to your kids' soccer games, keep singing with the choir, and keep having your parents over for lunch. Keep walking your dog or feeding the wild birds. Animals don't no-tice if you look funny or are less lively than you were, and those who know you make allowances. Social interaction encourages you to focus on other people and activities—something other than your own disrupted life. Doing things you enjoy or are good at establishes a continuity that counteracts feelings of disruption and loss. When you switch the spotlight away from yourself, help someone else, or solve a shared problem, you stop being a victim and become an ac-tor in life again. And being an actor restores your self-esteem.

You could decide to join a lupus support group and by sharing your problems help yourself and maybe others. Organizations and websites listed in Resources, at the end of the book, will help you find a group near you.

Give Yourself Rewards

Make a list of things you enjoy. Doing so is difficult when you are low, and at first you may have to enlist help. Maybe your partner will remind you, "Remember how much you laughed at *Shrek?*" Rent the video. Laughter is therapeutic. Write down favorite foods, favorite places, favorite simple pleasures: stroking the cat, burning scented candles, soaking in long, hot baths. Find little ways to reward yourself that will lift your spirits when you are down. Listing them is a valuable exercise in itself by turning your attention toward positive, enjoyable experiences. With practice you can train yourself to *think* about good experiences as a way of driving out negative thoughts, especially if they keep you awake at night. If your imagination isn't up to picturing yourself lying on the beach or listening to a nightingale, get a tape of soothing sounds to help you drop off to sleep.

Accentuate the Positive

The principle behind *cognitive behavioral therapy* (CBT), one of the most successful forms of psychotherapy, is modifying how you think. Every situation can be interpreted in different ways. With practice you can turn negative thoughts backward, as though you were arguing with someone. "I so miss sunbathing" becomes "I'll cultivate a pale and elegant look." "I'm such a burden on everyone" becomes "I'm so lucky that everyone is so helpful." Again, at first you may need help, so start the argument with someone else, such as a counselor, partner, or friend. Once you get the idea, every negative thought becomes a challenge: How can I turn it into a positive one?

"Choosing What to Eat Has Become a Minefield"

Both lupus and lupus medication can upset your stomach. Furthermore, if you have a chronic disease it is more important than ever to eat sensibly. Finally, you may have to deal with allergies, or foods that appear to prompt a flare-up. Nevertheless, it is important not to put too much emphasis on the role of food in illness. The phrase "you are what you eat" is an exaggeration and has promoted many wrong ideas. It is possible to make yourself less healthy by eating too much of the wrong things, or too little of the right things, but with few exceptions—bacterial contamination, genuine allergies, or food intolerances—food is neither the cause of disease nor a cure for it.

Nevertheless, you will be bombarded by books, magazine articles, and sites on the Internet that promise instant response in your disease symptoms from the introduction or removal of some dietary element, quite possibly costing you big money. Take it all with a very large pinch of salt. (Don't take too much real salt because that could be bad for fluid retention and your blood pressure.) Studies of large numbers of people with lupus are the most reliable source of information. Still, you will not necessarily conform to the norm. People can be very passionate about food, and if you believe that one food is making you feel better or another causing you flare-ups, it will do no harm to follow your instincts.

How Many Calories?

Being overweight is not good for anyone, and especially people with inflamed joints, but apart from this general health proviso, there is little evidence that quantity of food affects lupus. There have been studies that suggested that fasting or a vegetarian diet might reduce arthritic symptoms, but the studies were not very well controlled. There is sounder evidence when it comes to individual foods.

Fats

Graham Hughes reports the case history of a seriously ill rheumatoid arthritis patient who was passionate about cheese; she ate it every day. As a test, they tried withdrawing her daily cheese ration, in fact *all* dairy foods, for seven weeks. To everyone's surprise, within weeks there was a clinical improvement, so much so that in six months they were able to reduce her medication to zero. Being true scientists, they decided that, to confirm the relationship between dairy products and symptoms, they should give her cheese again—what is called "rechallenging" the symptoms. They tested her with several known food antigens with no response, finally giving her the cheese protein *casein*. Sure enough, the following day she was rigid with severe arthritis that lasted some days. She is now a healthy ex–cheese eater.

The effects of various sorts of fats in the diet have been studied in detail over the past decade. (In very crude terms, saturated = dairy products/red meat = bad, and unsaturated = fish = good.) Fats are thought to affect the autoimmune system via their action on the prostaglandins that cause inflammation. A study in which people with lupus reduced their total fat intake to 25 percent or less of their total daily caloric intake, which also included a fish-oil supplement, improved their symptoms over a three-month period. The explanation is thought to be that foods with *antioxidant* and anti-inflammatory properties lessen arthritic symptoms. One of these, the latest star in the nutrition galaxy, is omega-3 fatty acid, present in fish oils and some plant oils, including walnut, almond, flaxseed, and canola (rapeseed). It has been shown to reduce the pain and swelling of autoimmune arthritis.

Vitamins

Fish oil is also rich in vitamin D, thought to have anti-inflammatory properties. Studies support the idea that vitamin D, which the body needs to absorb calcium, has a protective role in arthritis and also helps to reduce the osteoporosis caused by using corticosteroids. Bearing in mind that vitamin D is obtainable chiefly from sunlight, which lupus sufferers must avoid, supplementing the vitamin via the diet makes a lot of sense. In addition to vitamin D, there is some evidence that a shortage of vitamin A may aggravate autoimmunity.

A Lupus-Drug Diet

Diet is a very important way to counteract the effects of lupus medication. You have already been warned about steroids; the list of potential damage they can cause, especially when taken in high doses and over long periods, makes very depressing reading, but even aspirin has a nutritional sting in its tail: It depletes vitamins A and

B-complex. Diuretics and some NSAIDs can also do damage, and all lupus medication carries a risk of upsetting digestion and damaging the lining of the digestive tract. But let's be positive: You can compensate for these hazards with the right diet.

General Rules

Take your drugs with food to decrease the irritating effect on the gut and to increase the time available for absorption of the drug. Avoid excess fluid, limit saturated fats (from dairy and red meat), and eat plenty of fiber, fruits, and vegetables to keep your weight down. Eat protein in moderation: meat sparingly (especially red meat), shellfish cautiously (oysters are a no-no for many lupus sufferers, and see the discussion of scallops in "Yellow-Light Foods," below), but fish in quantity, especially when you have a fever, which can cause nitrogen losses.

Green-Light Foods

To counteract the effect of lupus medication you need to boost potassium, calcium, zinc, iron, and vitamins A, B-complex and B-6, C, D, and E. Fortunately these double up in a number of foods: fruit (especially bananas for potassium, oranges and strawberries for vitamin C), plums, blackberries, avocado, and melon; vegetables, especially green ones such as broccoli, spinach, cauliflower, and green beans (with the exception of alfalfa sprouts; see page 88); oily fish like salmon, herring, tuna, and mackerel; high-fiber carbohydrates like whole-grain cereals, bread, nuts, and potatoes.

Yellow-Light Foods

Saturated fats—such as dairy products and fatty meats—should appear in your diet in moderation or low-fat versions. Eggs, like meat and dairy foods, are high in cholesterol and should therefore keep a low profile; so are scallops, but for most people they are too expensive and filling to eat in large quantities anyway.

Red-Light Foods

Eat as little salt as is palatable; it increases fluid retention and can raise blood pressure. Mushrooms, cured meats, and hot dogs should be consumed with caution. They contain chemicals that have been found to aggravate lupus symptoms (also see oysters, above).

Valerie's Story

Valerie, a lupus sufferer, was very positive about modifying her diet. As she puts it, "I lost twenty-four pounds by reducing fat and increasing my intake of vitamins and potassium (fruits like bananas and oranges). I have fewer pains in my knees because of this weight loss, and the vitamins seem to reduce the butterfly rash on my face. Who knows if diet helps lupus, but if you carry too many pounds the pain is certainly greater. And now I feel better with other people, because I feel pretty in my new body. It's a morale booster."

Are There No Alternatives?

Whenever a chronic illness that affects many people is inadequately controlled by orthodox medicine, you find a mushroom growth of alternative cures. It represents the capitalist marketing instinct responding to a natural human desire to try any port in a storm. Doctors are skeptical about such cures because they don't have to undergo the rigorous clinical testing demanded of a prescription medicine. The word "natural" often used for such cures is little more than a word printed on the label. Many herbs and supplements—some Chinese medicines for example—contain potent ingredients (and ones that may interfere with prescribed and effective medication), but in unreliable quantities. Attempts to test the efficacy of such products are hampered by the fact that few have a consistent content from one batch to another. Investigations triggered by occasional cases of someone coming to serious harm after taking alternative products have revealed that they may contain substances not mentioned in the labeling, such as powerful hormones, potent anti-inflammatories with major side effects, or sulfa drugs that set off hypersensitivity reactions and react with other drugs. Lupus expert Sheldon Blau cites one supplement—alfalfa sprout—that, between the years 1995 and 2002, was associated with seventeen outbreaks of food poisoning caused by salmonella or *E. coli* infection (as reported to the U.S. Centers for Disease Control and Prevention). People with lupus are particularly vulnerable because they are at greater than average risk of suffering hypersensitive or allergic reactions to something like St. John's wort, which can trigger severe photosensitivity.

Suffice to say that as a lupus sufferer you should be hypercautious about what you swallow—whether in the form of so-called alternative cures or food supplements—because you cannot be absolutely sure of what's in them. If in doubt, don't take it.

Therapies That May Help

Treat your digestive system with respect, but the outside of your body may indeed benefit from therapies not provided by orthodox medicine or physiotherapy. Relaxation and exercise techniques like yoga, t'ai chi, acupuncture, meditation, and aromatherapy are undoubtedly stress reducing and psychologically beneficial for a large number of chronic or incurable conditions. Acupuncture has demonstrated some painkilling effects. Many people with lupus, not to mention the unaffected, swear by them. A study of patients in North America and the United Kingdom, published in the journal *Arthritis and Rheumatism*, found that nearly half had tried alternative therapies. If you think you have found something that helps you and which doesn't clobber your bank account, it does no harm, provided you don't stop your prescribed medication.

Chapter 9

Seven Lupus-Like
Conditions

Lupus, as we have seen, is exceedingly difficult to pin down. It comes and goes, and in many guises. For years it was thought to be more than one disease, and even now the boundaries between lupus and lupus-like conditions are constantly shifting. The labeling of illnesses is an imperfect science and is always under review.

The majority of people with lupus have lupus alone. Between 5 and 30 percent of people with lupus have overlapping symptoms. Connective tissue diseases (CTDs), a category that includes lupus and rheumatoid arthritis, are particularly prone to this overlap phenomenon. Conditions like Raynaud's phenomenon or Sjögren's syndrome may put in an appearance with lupus or a number of CTDs and may also occur alone. (Some of these conditions have already been mentioned and will be familiar to the reader.) Establishing what an individual patient is suffering from ultimately lands in the lap of the diagnosing physician. Fortunately, treatment is driven by individual clinical symptoms, so it does not vary greatly.

CTDs have a number of features in common:

▶ They affect women much more frequently than men.

▶ They are "multisystem": They affect the function of many organs.

▶ They overlap with one another, sharing symptoms, signs, and abnormalities detected in the laboratory.

▶ Blood vessels are the most common target of injury.

▶ The abnormal behavior of the immune system is responsible, at least in part, for the tissue damage they cause.

This chapter examines some of the illnesses whose symptoms can overlap with those of lupus.

Mixed Connective Tissue Disease (MCTD)

To the layperson this mouthful of a title probably seems a bit of an evasion. Graham Hughes calls it a "mongrel" because it combines symptoms of lupus with those of other CTDs (see Chapter 1 and Chapter 4). It may include:

▶ Arthritis (especially of the hands—"sausage fingers")

▶ Polymyositis-dermatomyositis, or PM-DM (muscle inflammation)

▶ Scleroderma (hardening of the skin or connective tissue)

▶ Raynaud's phenomenon (poor circulation leading to very cold extremities)

What distinguishes MCTD from lupus pure and simple is that it is almost never accompanied by the involvement of organs like the kidneys. Laboratory tests usually reveal that the patient has one specific antibody called "antiRNP" but none of the other antibodies commonly associated with lupus, scleroderma, or PM-DM. Although there is some doubt as to whether MCTD really is a separate disease or several diseases showing up together in the same patient, the presence of the single antibody weights the scales in favor of a distinct disease.

MCTD treatment is geared to the symptoms experienced by the individual patient. But because the condition is less life-threatening than lupus or rheumatoid arthritis, doctors tend to be as conservative as possible in prescribing drugs. Nevertheless, low to moderate doses of steroids are often required for many years to control MCTD adequately.

Raynaud's phenomenon—another condition named after the doctor who first described it—may occur either as part of MCTD, in conjunction with lupus (between 20 and 40 percent of cases), or alone (between 5 and 10 percent of the population). It's caused by a sudden constriction of the smallest arteries, cutting off the peripheral circulation, an exaggerated version of the body's normal response to extreme cold and the need to conserve heat. In addition to practical measures, such as keeping the hands and feet well insulated in cold weather (some people use electrically heated gloves), drugs that relax and dilate blood vessels can be helpful. Calcium antagonists, which were originally designed to lower blood pressure and treat coronary heart disease, have been found particularly beneficial. Some doctors prefer to prescribe regular, low-dose aspirin as a preventative. This is also protective against coronary artery disease and stroke.

Sjögren's Syndrome

Henrik Sjögren (the nearest pronunciation is "showgrin") was a Swedish ophthalmologist and the first to recognize that people with CTDs often had dry eyes and mouth, or sicca (dry) syndrome (see Chapter 4). The dryness is caused by a buildup of immune system cells in and around glands that produce tears and saliva, leading to reduced production of these essential fluids. Some 5 percent of lupus patients develop Sjögren's, sometimes late in life when most of their other symptoms have abated. The eyes feel gritty and itchy, especially early in the morning, and sometimes they are also sensitive to bright light. But discomfort is not the only symptom. Tears and saliva perform an important protective function, and without them the eyes and teeth are more prone to infection. Saliva normally helps wash away plaque, the invisible bacterial film that develops on the surface of tooth enamel and leads to cavities and gum disease. A diagnosis of Sjögren's is extremely difficult; it has been known to take as long as two or even eight years! Meanwhile, treatment is necessarily symptomatic. A special low-concentration eyewash containing cyclosporine, a powerful immunosuppressant, may be prescribed, or an oral antimalarial like hydroxychloroquine. For dry mouth, prescription drugs are available that stimulate the production of saliva, for example pilocarpine (Salagen). Regular dental checkups are vital. There are also mechanical topical treatments for the eyes, in the form of drops called "artificial tears" (which are usually satisfactory), and for the mouth, in the form of "artificial saliva" sprays (which are usually not satisfactory). It is possible to block the tear ducts surgically to retain moisture, and of course sufferers need to avoid smoke, strong winds, and any form of airborne irritant, and to use eye makeup extremely sparingly. Sufferers should beware of proprietary over-the-counter products that promise to cure sore, reddened eyes. These contain *vasoconstrictors* that make blood vessels constrict, aggravating the dryness and discomfort of Sjögren's. For more information on Sjögren's syndrome and how to cope with it, I recommend Sue Dyson's *Positive Options for Sjögren's Syndrome* (see Further Reading).

Fibromyalgia

Fibromyalgia, or fibromyalgia syndrome (FMS), was only recognized by the American College of Rheumatology (ACR) and included in the official diagnostic manuals in 1990. The name derives from three Greek root words—*fibro-* (fibrous or connective tissue), *my-* (muscle), *algos* (pain)—but its most prominent symptom is debilitating fatigue. Some experts believe it is the same condition known as chronic fatigue syndrome, now usually called myalgic encephalitis or ME (more Greek, meaning "brain inflammation").

Characteristically, the pain of FMS is spread throughout the body, not confined to joints. In addition, people with FMS may experience disturbed sleep patterns, difficulty in concentrating, migraine headaches, anxiety and depression, hearing and seeing problems, and heart-valve abnormalities (see the box "A Hole-in-the-Heart Link to Headaches," below). Things are usually worse in the morning. Some studies suggest that sufferers may also have unusual variations in hormonal or other biochemical patterns, and some also suffer from Raynaud's phenomenon. Brain-imaging technology confirms that FMS sufferers actually process pain signals differently from most people; their pain is amplified, as though the volume has been turned up. For more information on FMS, I recommend Katrina Berne's *Chronic Fatigue Syndrome, Fibromyalgia and Other Invisible Illnesses* (see Further Reading).

> ### A Hole-in-the-Heart Link to Headaches
>
> Thousands of migraine sufferers, including many of those diagnosed with FMS or ME, may have a small hole in the heart that can be corrected by a simple patch. A clinical trial currently in progress is investigating those who suffer from severe migraine accompanied by pins-and-needles and by a visual disturbance known as aura: flashing lights, bright spots, blind spots, or like seeing through a snowstorm. Research suggests that as many as 17 percent of migraine sufferers may fall into this category. Researchers believe that these migraine sufferers may have a common heart defect called patent formen ovale (PFO), shared with up to a quarter of the population, the majority totally unaware. A PFO is a hole, usually harmless, up to a centimeter across, located between the two upper chambers of the heart. The researchers believe that in these cases some blood that should be filtered through the lungs may bypass them through the PFO, allowing chemicals that contribute to migraine to get to the brain.
>
> The connection between holes in the heart and headaches was discovered serendipitously when a number of migraine sufferers who were among stroke victims and deep-sea divers with "the bends" underwent the patch procedure to correct their PFOs and discovered that their headaches also disappeared.

Like the other disorders described in this chapter, FMS can exist alone or with one or more CTDs. Up to a third of those with a CTD, including lupus, may have it. As with nearly all these conditions, the cause is unknown. There is some evidence of familial, probably genetic predisposition, with the likely trigger being a virus or other infection. Treatment is again targeted on symptoms. Unlike lupus, FMS does not respond to steroids, antimalarials, or immunosuppressants, and NSAIDs are usually inadequate in the face of the severe pain, which may demand stronger painkilling drugs called *opiates*. Sometimes antidepressants seem to relieve the pain: either an older tricyclic drug called amitriptyline (Elavil) or one of the newer selective serotonin reuptake inhibitors (SSRIs, e.g., Prozac). These are usually given in lower doses than are required for anxiety or depression. Trials are going on to see if an antiseizure drug, gabapentin (Neurontin), which has been successful in reducing various sorts of nerve pain, might be effective in treating FMS.

To date the most successful ways of treating FMS are through self-help techniques. Sufferers learn to avoid extremes of cold or heat; physical or mental stress; and either too much or, conversely, too little exercise. Living in a climate with warm, dry weather is ideal. And the best physical activities seem to be things like regular, gentle cycling on flat surfaces, t'ai chi, gentle stretching, and swimming in a heated pool. A physiotherapist may be able to devise a routine for FMS sufferers. Professional massage and acupuncture have helped some people.

Libman-Sacks Endocarditis

Two more American physicians bequeathed their names to posterity in 1923 by describing a condition that is estimated to affect from 10 to 20 percent of people with lupus.

In Chapter 1, I explained that the sheaths that line the heart and lungs are made of connective tissue and are therefore vulnerable in lupus and other CTDs. Pericarditis, inflammation of the lining of the heart, is relatively common in lupus. *Endocarditis* involves the interior of the heart (*endo* is Greek for "inside"), in particular, the valves between chambers that regulate the flow of blood and prevent it from going the wrong way. In Libman-Sacks endocarditis (LSE), tiny wartlike growths develop on the valves, causing them to leak. Most people who develop it also have antiphospholipid antibodies (APS, or Hughes' syndrome, introduced in Chapter 5 and dealt with in detail in Chapter 10).

Doctors detect the possibility of LSE from listening to the heart (see box "Listening to the Heart," below). Heart valves affected by LSE cause a distinctive type of murmur behind the sound of the heartbeat. If the doctor thinks he or she can hear it, he or she will probably confirm suspicions by asking the hospital to do an *echocardiograph*. Echocardiography passes sound waves into the chest, where they are reflected back to the instrument from the solid structures inside, providing an "echo" of the structure. The instrument forms a picture of the heart structure from the reflected sound waves; it is the same principle as radar or bats' sonar.

Listening to the Heart

What does a family doctor, or indeed a cardiologist, hear when he or she sticks the stethoscope on your chest?

The heart is a synchronized pump—or, if you prefer, a pair of pumps, synchronized to pass blood between their chambers and push it through the lungs and around the body. The skilled listener hears the one-way valves opening and shutting and blood being driven from one chamber in the heart to another. There are four distinct sounds in a normal heartbeat, usually described as making a noise rather like "lop-dop." The explosive consonants in "lop-dop" are made by the valves opening and closing. A doctor learns to detect the sound of a healthy heart even though there may be slight variations in the patterns of sound. The doctor will note the speed of the beat. Does the heart race, or even gallop? He or she may also hear noises in between the distinct beats of the heart. These are called murmurs, and may indicate that the various valves are not working properly, for example, leaking and allowing some blood to go the wrong way.

These days there are many sophisticated ways of assessing the heart's performance: by plotting electrical impulses from the heart muscle (electrocardiogram), by constructing images of the blood flow (magnetic resonance imaging or MRI), or by analyzing the sounds (echocardiograph). The stethoscope applied to the medically trained ear dominates front-line diagnosis because it is portable and doesn't need to be plugged in.

In itself LSE is not dangerous. Problems arise if the warts grow-ing on the valves become infected. Various things can cause this but the most common is dental treatment. The mouth is a veritable hotbed of bacteria. And bacteria may get into the bloodstream if the body's internal mucous lining is broken during dental proce-dures or during medical procedures such as undergoing a cervical smear or a *colonoscopy* (an internal investigation of the colon using a fiber-optic camera).

If an infection does occur in the heart valves the symptoms are fever, irregular heartbeat, difficulty breathing, and, if not treated, heart failure. To avoid this risk, LSE sufferers are prescribed antibi-otics as a precautionary measure in advance of any risky dental or medical procedure.

Avascular Necrosis

Avascular necrosis is the exception to the general rule that lupus, un-like rheumatoid arthritis, is not progressive and does not do perma-nent damage to joints. (See box "Cell Death and Recycling," on the facing page.)

Joint pain is a feature of lupus for many. A small number also suffer actual damage to some part of the joint. The condition is known by a variety of names, most of which describe what it is *not*. It is not damage caused by trauma (atraumatic); it is not damage caused by infection (aseptic); what it is caused by is reduced blood supply, hence the name *avascular* necrosis. (Diminished blood sup-ply leads to shortage of red blood cells, hence disruption to the de-livery of their oxygen payload, and hence tissue damage.) There is uncertainty about how many lupus sufferers experience joint necro-sis; it may be as many as 40 percent, or it may be as few as 5 percent.

Two parts of the joint may be damaged by avascular necrosis. First, bone, particularly the head of the bone in load-bearing joints like the hips, knees, and shoulders. (These are frequently the sites of other forms of arthritis, both wear-and-tear osteoarthritis and rheumatoid arthritis.) When bone is affected the condition may be

> **Cell Death and Recycling**
>
> For animals, death is the end. If it comes during sleep, in the fullness of years, it is reckoned slightly better than if the animal is cut off in its prime, but it is still the end. It is a little different with cells. Cells are what living organisms are composed of, whether a tree, a goldfish, or your old Uncle Harry, and they come and go in a constant cycle throughout the lifetime of the organism. It's as though Uncle Harry were a waterfall. (Don't be difficult; just try to imagine it.) The water in the waterfall is always changing, but the waterfall itself is still the same waterfall. That's how it is with the cells of the body. They are continuously produced (give or take a few exceptions like the corneal surface of the eye and some brain cells), go about their business, and then die off in an orderly and preprogrammed manner to get reabsorbed into the body—a sort of cell recycling. This end is known in medicine as apoptosis. You have met it in connection with the cells of the immune system, some of which fail to do this in autoimmune diseases.
>
> *Necrosis* is a Greek word for "death." (You may recognize this root in words like necropolis, a place where the dead are buried, or necrophilia, a disturbed erotic obsession with a dead person or people.) The term "necrosis" is used in medicine to describe unscheduled and unhealthy death of cells or some part of the body—cell death as decay.

called *osteonecrosis,* adding the Greek term for "bone" to "necrosis." Second, many more lupus patients suffer damage to tendons (the cable-like structures that tether muscle to bone) caused by disrupted blood supply. This is known as tendon rupture, but is also described as "fraying" or "tearing." The affected tendon does not need to be load-bearing, and the most common site is the fingers. The rupture causes a sudden collapse of the bone supported by the tendon and can be quite alarming. If it is one of the bones of the hands, the person may drop something; if it is a leg tendon, he or she may fall down. One patient described it by saying, "I've severed tendons like they were spaghetti, including the tendons in both of my thumbs—one of them twice. The latest was a *patellar tendon* in my knee. It happens when I am doing quite simple things; with one of my thumbs I was just picking up a bag of oranges! I've had more surgery than anybody I know."

Lupus patients with a history of arthritis, blood disorders like anemia, circulatory problems, high blood pressure, elevated cholesterol, diabetes, heavy drinking or (perish the thought) smoking are more at risk for avascular necrosis. If bone is affected (the previously mentioned osteonecrosis) the first symptom is likely to be pain in the joint itself, or possibly pain referred to a nearby area. If the necrosis is not checked, there may also be pain at rest. Without treatment the necrosis causes actual loss of tissue in the joint, leading to collapse and fracture. At first, the damage does not show up on X rays, though it does on more sensitive imaging technologies.

Hopefully, early intervention will prevent necrosis from progressing to this point. The first-line treatment, once the problem is detected, is with drugs. In fact, patients identified as being at high risk are usually offered prophylactic (preventive) treatment to head off even the possibility of joint damage. Some risk factors can be reduced by modifying the lifestyle (cutting out cigarettes, alcohol, and fatty junk foods), and others, like high blood pressure, anemia, and elevated cholesterol, can be treated with relatively side effect–free drugs. If bone damage is detected early, a surgical procedure called *core decompression* will be recommended. Under anesthetic, a small core of tissue is withdrawn from inside the blood-deprived area of bone to relieve the pressure and also to encourage the formation of new, fine blood vessels and healthy bone. This procedure has been in use for more than thirty years and has a good record of helping patients avoid more radical surgical treatment.

Once osteonecrosis reaches the stage at which it shows up on X-ray images, core decompression may be too late. Replacing the affected joint may then be necessary, especially in the case of a load-bearing joint like the hip or knee. This may sound radical, but it has become an almost routine procedure for many people with osteoarthritis (the common wear-and-tear kind). Artificial knee and hip replacements have a very satisfactory history of restored movement and reduced pain. Ruptured tendons also have to be repaired by surgery.

Drug-Induced Lupus (DIL)

This last lupus-like condition is not so much a lamb dressed up as a wolf as it is a completely human-made wolf. To be precise, this is an *iatrogenic* form of lupus, meaning it is caused by doctors or medical treatment (*iatros* is Greek for "physician"). As one doctor puts it, "Iatrogenic basically means it's our fault."

Mitch's Story

Like a number of men who had worked hard, lived well, and not gotten enough exercise, Mitch's blood pressure crept up in middle age. High blood pressure increases the chances of heart disease and stroke, and a good doctor always insists on correcting it. In Mitch's case modifying the lifestyle—cutting out salt, soft-pedalling the booze, and getting out onto the golf course more—didn't achieve adequate results. What's more, at one of his regular checkups, his physician discovered that he had an irregular heartbeat, one of the early signs of heart disease. She prescribed a drug to bring down the blood pressure and another to stabilize the heartbeat. At first, things improved, and so did Mitch's handicap.

Some months later Mitch began to suffer from extreme fatigue. The cardiologist whom he was seeing told him to get more exercise. "How can I get more exercise when I feel exhausted from the moment I wake up," he complained to his wife. And then one morning he fell over at the first tee. His leg just gave way beneath him. He got up and tried to go on, but a few yards farther down the fairway his other leg gave out. He went to his family doctor. She did a thorough examination and discovered that he was suffering from muscle weakness in both legs. His muscles were wasting away. She took blood and told Mitch she thought he had developed DIL. She stopped the drugs he had been taking and prescribed known, safe alternatives. She also sent Mitch off to a physiotherapist for a course of exercise to build up his wasted muscles.

More than one hundred different drugs have been reported as causing lupus-like conditions (see box "Some Drugs That Induce Lupus Symptoms," below). The phenomenon was first noted in the 1940s. We know that some drugs (antibiotics, for example) can cause a flare in someone who already has lupus, but these drugs cause it in otherwise lupus-free people. The two drugs Mitch reacted to are those most often implicated, though they are not prescribed frequently these days.

Some Drugs That Induce Lupus Symptoms

▶ Hydralazine (blood-pressure lowering agent)

▶ Procainamide, quinidine bisulfate (for irregular heart rhythm)

▶ Sulfasalazine (anti-inflammatory used for colitis and rheumatoid arthritis)

▶ Minocycline (antibiotic used for acne)

▶ Penicillamine (antibiotic)

▶ Isoniazid (antibiotic used for tuberculosis)

▶ Chlorpromazine (used for serious mental illness and severe nausea)

▶ Methyldopa (used for Parkinson's disease)

▶ Phenytoin (an anticonvulsant, used for epilepsy)

Some of the very latest drugs, for example biological agents developed to treat rheumatoid arthritis, have also been implicated in drug-induced lupus.

What's the difference between drug-induced lupus (DIL) and the genuine article? Symptoms are usually, though not invariably, less severe; there may be fatigue, arthritis, widespread rashes, swollen lymph glands, pleurisy, or pericarditis, but it is rare for the condition to cause kidney damage. Blood tests do not reveal the characteristic pattern of antibodies, but reveal some similarities and some differences, depending on the drug culprit causing the trouble. The principle difference is that all symptoms disappear soon after the drugs are withdrawn, leaving no lasting damage.

In the United States, as many as fifty thousand people are thought to suffer from DIL, though Graham Hughes says that in his experience it is "rare" in the U.K. Clearly the incidence of any iatrogenic condition is not a natural phenomenon. If the at-risk people and culprit drugs can be positively identified, there should ideally be zero cases to report. However, it is not absolutely clear why some people develop DIL with certain drugs. One theory holds that some people metabolize drugs more slowly and may therefore be more vulnerable. It seems likely, as with lupus itself, that some genetic factor contributes to lupus being triggered by drugs.

Chapter 10

Lupus and Pregnancy

History provides us with a dramatic example of the effect lupus can have upon childbearing.

Queen Anne's Story

Queen Anne, of England, died in 1714, tormented as much by her physicians' misguided efforts at treatment as by her own agonizing illness. Her short life had been plagued by ill health, not least by an exhausting succession of miscarriages. In the first eighteen years of her marriage she had seventeen pregnancies, including eleven miscarriages, and only one child survived infancy. Since one of her primary aims in life, as the last of the Stuart line, a dynasty plagued by religious strife for nearly a hundred years, was to produce a Protestant heir, this was a bitter failure.

In his book *The Sickly Stuarts*, Professor Fredrick Holmes, of the University of Kansas Medical Center, writes, "Systemic lupus erythematosus remains the best explanation for Anne's ill-starred obstetric history and the disabling rheumatic disease she suffered in the last decade or so of her life ... which led to her premature death from a cerebrovascular event—a stroke—common among sufferers of this disease."

In the views of both Professor Holmes and Graham Hughes, Anne had lupus with antiphospholipid antibody syndrome (APS), a blood condition that, unchecked, causes pregnancies to fail at between three and five months because of thrombosis: blood clots blocking the small blood vessels to the placenta, which feeds the fetus. In modern times, if the antibody is identified, a single aspirin a day can prevent miscarriage. Reflecting on this remedy Professor Holmes writes, "In all likelihood in the early eighteenth century the equivalent was actually available as salicylic acid in herbal preparations containing willow bark, although its efficacy in Anne's condition could not have been known at the time.... [C]learly Anne had the antiphospholipid antibody."

If Queen Anne's doctors had known what we know today, history might have followed a different course; the house of Hanover might not have inherited the throne of England, and George III might not have lost the American colonies!

As recently as twenty-five years ago, doctors usually advised women with lupus not to get pregnant because recurrent miscarriage was a known symptom of the disease. But with a better understanding of the reasons behind these miscarriages the picture has changed. Studies of lupus pregnancies reveal that, whereas forty years ago less than half of them resulted in live births, these days between two-thirds and three-quarters are successful. And these figures are averages; in some hospitals, what is known as the "take-home-baby" rate is even higher, although in about a quarter of lupus pregnancies there remains a risk of premature birth.

Facing Up to the Risks

Among the barrage of laboratory tests lupus patients undergo during diagnosis is one that is central to the outcome of pregnancy: the test for APS, an illness we discussed in Chapter 5. APS is now recognized as a distinct autoimmune disease in its own right, but whereas only about 5 percent of the general population exhibit it, a very high percentage of lupus sufferers do. It is associated with increased risk of the formation of obstructive blood clots, which in turn increase the danger of heart attack or stroke and, when they obstruct the blood supply to the placenta, which nourishes the fetus, starve it of oxygen and cause miscarriage. The syndrome was first identified by Graham Hughes, of St. Thomas' Hospital, London, and is also known as Hughes' syndrome. (See Graham Hughes' book on lupus or Triona Holden's *Positive Options for Living with Antiphospholipid Syndrome (APS)* in "Further Reading.")

People with APS often have a wide range of other symptoms— seizures, migraine, joint pain and inflammation, avascular necrosis (see Chapter 9), leg ulcers, anemia—most of them traceable to problems with circulation and thrombosis. All APS-related difficulties are made worse by smoking, high blood pressure, diabetes, and high levels of cholesterol and other *lipids* (soluble fats) in the bloodstream.

Two further antibodies can cause trouble in pregnancy. One is called *anticardiolipin* (ACL), and the other is lupus anticoagulant (LAC). These two work in different ways to increase problems with circulation and heart function, and to increase the risk of miscarriage.

A diagnosis of APS requires both clinical symptoms—thrombosis or a history of miscarriage—and positive laboratory tests for ACL or LAC. As with other autoimmune diseases, the cause of APS is unknown, though studies support the idea of a genetic susceptibility triggered by a viral infection.

Any woman who is undertaking a pregnancy and is diagnosed with APS, including those who also have lupus, will be put on an aggressive pharmaceutical regime to correct the condition: drugs to lower high blood pressure, high cholesterol, and other blood lipids, and also to control diabetes. The risk of blood clots can be reduced by prescribing aspirin or more powerful "blood-thinning" drugs such as heparin.

It goes without saying that she will also be adjured to strictly follow rigid pregnancy health behaviors. She shouldn't smoke or drink, or dabble with "recreational" drugs or any pharmacy product or supplement not prescribed by her doctor. She should pay particular attention to eating a balanced diet, follow her prescribed lupus medication to the letter, and, above all, stay in close contact with her rheumatologist as well as her obstetrician. Keeping lupus and APS under control during the pregnancy is absolutely central.

The medical team will inevitably rule out a home delivery. Women with lupus—or women with any chronic condition that poses a risk to either mother or child—need to be in a good hospital under a specialist's care when they give birth. There is an ever-present risk of premature birth with a lupus pregnancy, and that dictates having access to a unit equipped to care for the premature, or otherwise distressed, newborn.

Lupus Drugs During Pregnancy

It goes against instinct to be taking powerful drugs during pregnancy. And some drugs prescribed for lupus are indeed contraindicated, but surprisingly few. Steroids, probably prednisolone, even in quite large doses, do not appear to do harm. The mother's body breaks down this drug in the placenta in such a way that limits the amount reaching the fetus, though it is important that taking it doesn't lead to the mother's gaining excessive weight. Some steroids do cross the placental barrier and may be used deliberately when an effect on the baby is intended. If a premature birth looks likely, a steroid called dextramethasone may be given to accelerate the development of the baby's lungs and reduce the breathing problems babies suffer when born early.

In the past, antimalarials have been withdrawn during pregnancy because they cross the placental barrier, but a recent French study suggests that possibly hydroxychloroquine may after all be safe, although a full examination of the eyes of the babies born in the study (vision is at risk from antimalarials) has not yet been completed. Powerful immunosuppressants are also usually avoided, although Graham Hughes reports that as many as fifteen hundred lupus patients in the U.K. achieved successful pregnancies while on azathioprine. It is probably safer to say that the jury is still out on both drugs.

The immunosuppressant cyclophosphamide is definitely off limits, as are the blood-pressure drugs known as *ACE inhibitors,* which can harm the baby if taken in the last six months of the pregnancy. (Other blood-pressure drugs can be substituted.) The anticoagulant (blood-thinning) drug warfarin, which can harm the embryo in early pregnancy, is also ruled out. Heparin is the preferred alternative.

Pregnancy and childbirth, of course, involve massive changes to hormone levels in a woman's body. It would be surprising if pregnancy didn't have some effect upon a condition like lupus, which is known to be highly sensitive to the balance between various hormones. Even the most scrupulous care in monitoring the mother's health during pregnancy may fail to avoid a slight increase in the number of flares she experiences, but in general these are mild and easily controlled. There's a greater chance of a flare-up immediately after delivery, when she experiences a sudden drop in progesterone, the hormone that has helped to maintain the pregnancy. To counter this effect, some doctors increase the dosage of steroids around the start of labor, gradually tapering it off only weeks after the birth. Others prefer to increase steroids only if and when a flare-up occurs. This is because at the time of birth it's important to consider what drugs may get into the mother's milk and so affect the baby. Breastfeeding has such wide-ranging benefits for the baby that the obstetric team does everything to make it easy for a new mother to breastfeed. And this may mean, shortly before the baby arrives, reducing drugs like antimalarials or aspirin that have helped keep the pregnancy flare-free. Once again, steroids do not pose a problem.

Risks to the Baby

The biggest risk to a lupus birth is that it may occur too soon. As mentioned, even with advanced, modern treatment about a quarter of lupus births are premature. These days, hospitals' premature-baby units are so sophisticated that we have become almost blasé about the problem, but it is still the goal of all good obstetricians that mothers go to full term, that is, between thirty-five and thirty-seven weeks, or at the very least until the baby weighs three and a half pounds. Premature babies have difficulty controlling their body temperature (and therefore have to spend a period in an incubator); they are also likely to have problems breathing because their lungs are not fully developed, or to have difficulty sucking. At the very least, prematurity risks interfering with the bonding between mother and child that develops with established breastfeeding.

A number of risk factors common to all pregnancies can be more problematic for a lupus mother. One is a condition known as *preeclampsia*, or toxemia of pregnancy, which occurs when the kidneys, overwhelmed by the extra work of filtering the blood supply for an additional person, fail to eliminate all the waste products they usually clear from the bloodstream. Preeclampsia occurs late in pregnancy and is signaled by a rise in blood pressure, the presence of protein in the urine (normally filtered out by the kidneys), and edema (fluid retention) that causes puffy ankles, fingers, and knees—another sign that the kidneys are not working well.

As you might deduce, preeclampsia is the prelude to a condition called eclampsia, which is fortunately extremely rare these days because the warning signs are usually detected. It occurs when the inability of the kidneys to clear fluid from the tissues leads to seizures, unconsciousness, and even possibly death. Regular monitoring of blood pressure and urine normally picks up the danger signals in time, and since the delivery date is usually not far away, the doctors typically decide to induce birth or even to perform a Caesarean section. Left unchecked, the condition threatens the lives of both mother and child. Preeclampsia is a complication that affects between 5 and 7 percent of all pregnancies but about 20 percent of lupus pregnancies.

One other risk factor affects lupus pregnancies more than others. At about the fourteenth week of pregnancy the obstetrician usually tests the mother's blood for *alphafetoprotein (AFP)*. This is made almost exclusively by the baby's liver, and it is quite normal for levels to increase to some degree. However, exceptionally high concentrations seem to be associated with serious abnormalities of the baby's brain and spinal cord called *neural-tube defects (NTD)*. Only a minority of babies born following elevated AFP go on to develop NTD, but it is important that lupus mothers be monitored because they are more likely to develop high concentrations. The good news is that this doesn't seem to reflect a higher than normal chance that their babies will have NTD; rather it seems related to the increased risk of those babies arriving prematurely. It also seems to go with higher doses of prednisolone—possibly for women with less well-controlled lupus.

Will the Baby Be All Right?

You can see that in getting pregnant a woman with lupus is undertaking something that, while less hazardous than it was forty years ago, is nevertheless not risk-free. The questions all parents ask, including those without lupus, are: Will nine months of caution and careful monitoring produce the hoped-for reward? Will we have a healthy baby at the end of this pregnancy?

Lupus, as explained, is not directly inherited from mother to child. What does sometimes happen is that babies born to lupus mothers develop a short-lived, lupus-related condition called *neonatal* lupus. Up to the moment of birth, mother and baby have exchanged blood through the placenta, and what seems to happen is that some lupus antibodies have snuck across the placenta and gotten stranded in the baby, where they inflame the baby's skin. Almost invariably the culprits are anti-Ro antibodies (a subset of ANA antibodies). Between 30 and 40 percent of lupus patients have anti-Ro antibodies, and between 10 and 20 percent of mothers with the antibodies give birth to babies who exhibit neonatal lupus. At most we're talking about 8 percent of all lupus mothers. But the situation gives the new mother quite a scare because the baby develops a butterfly rash.

It must be emphasized that this condition is rare. Graham Hughes, who has seen thousands of lupus mothers through pregnancy, says he has only seen about a dozen cases in all his professional life. And it isn't real lupus. It's just a dying echo of the mother's lupus, and it quickly clears up as the mother's antibodies disappear from the baby's blood.

Occasionally (in less than half the cases of neonatal lupus) the baby is born with a slight heart abnormality called *heart-block;* the electrical impulses of the heart are irregular, making it sound as though it is stopping. But it doesn't. In itself slight heart *arrhythmias* are not life-threatening. (In older people they can be a warning of something that *might* be life-threatening.) In a very few cases—we are now getting down to vanishingly small percentages—the baby's arrhythmia is serious enough to require a pacemaker.

For Those Who Don't Want to Get Pregnant

Dora's Story

Dora had a bad pregnancy in the early 1990s. She had blood clots and inflammation in the veins of her legs (thrombophlebitis) and fragments of blood clots in her lungs (pulmonary emboli). Her doctors advised her not to get pregnant again, so she started taking the contraceptive pill. Then she developed some weird, really painful red lumps on her legs. Her doctor was bewildered and referred her to a rheumatologist, who carried out blood tests. The rheumatologist told Dora that she had both lupus and APS. The lumps, she was told, were erythema nodosum (Greek for "red lumps"), a form of *vasculitis* not exclusive to lupus sufferers though more common among them, which occasionally appeared on other parts of the body. The rheumatologist took Dora off the pill and in its place recommended a diaphragm.

If a woman with lupus decides she would rather not get pregnant, what should she do? To all appearances, controlled lupus has no effect on fertility, although fertile periods are sometimes interrupted during a lupus flare-up. If she wants to avoid or plan pregnancy she needs some form of contraception. The female hormone estrogen is known to exacerbate lupus symptoms, and thus for twenty years the usual advice has been for lupus sufferers not to use the birth-control pill, especially those who experience the migraine and clotting problems associated with APS. However, a survey of patients at St. Thomas' Hospital found that the same proportion of female lupus patients were taking oral contraceptives as of nonlupus mothers, with no apparent increase of side effects. Then, at the end of 2004, the Safety of Estrogens in Systemic Lupus Erythematosus National Assessment (SELENA) study, conducted in the United States, reported similar results. Dr. Michelle Petri of Johns Hopkins Hospital told the annual scientific meeting of the American College of Rheumatology (ACR), "This is a clinical trial you can take home with you. It will change the way you practice." Henceforth, the trial concluded, oral contraceptives should be regarded as acceptable for the two-thirds of lupus patients who are not at risk of thrombosis. This is good news because women with lupus are at higher-than-average risk of osteoporosis as a consequence of taking steroids, and estrogen is known to protect against this condition.

Lupus patients who also have APS are still advised not to use any form of hormonal contraception—whether the pill, injections, patches, or implants—because they may aggravate circulatory problems, high blood pressure, vasculitis, and thrombosis. Some doctors believe that progestogen-only contraceptives are acceptable, but in general Sheldon Blau's advice remains: "Shun all forms of hormonal contraception." Intrauterine devices (IUDs) are also unsuitable for lupus patients because they have a higher likelihood of suffering perforation, bleeding, or pelvic infections with the device. For some female lupus patients, as you can see, it comes down to good old barrier contraceptives: the diaphragm and condoms. These, of course, however inconvenient they may seem, have the added advantage of protecting against sexually transmitted infection.

Chapter 11

Foretelling the Future

Hippocrates, ancient Greek physician and father of medicine, gave his pupils modest goals: to help, or at least to do no harm. His instruction comes not from the celebrated oath—still taken by many medical students today—but from another of his writings called the *Epidemics.* Translated in full it reads, "Declare the past, diagnose the present, foretell the future; practice these acts. As to diseases, make a habit of two things—to help, or at least to do no harm."

Modern physicians have more ambitious goals: to bring relief, to cure, and (the Holy Grail) wherever possible to prevent illness. In some cases—for example with childhood diseases and infections, and with diseases caused by dietary deficiency—they have had spectacular success. In the case of the many forms of arthritis their success has been confined to bringing relief, controlling symptoms, and preventing the worst damage. Cure is still a long way off; prevention even further.

As for the future, doctors' ability to predict medical outcomes has made rapid strides in modern times. Researchers believe that there is hope that their understanding of autoimmune diseases such as rheumatoid arthritis will provide greater control over outcomes in the not too distant future. Understanding opens the door to more precise, effective treatment, and side-effect-free treatment is the penultimate stop before cure. Prevention depends ultimately on understanding not only *what* goes wrong, but *why*, which, in the terms of the current hypothesis about autoimmune diseases, means identifying the triggers that set off the abnormal autoimmune reaction, and the genes that make some people susceptible in the first place. The answers, when they come, will probably emerge little by little, because it is possible that there will turn out to be more than one trigger, and certainly more than one susceptible gene.

This chapter looks into the crystal ball to see what shapes are emerging from the mist, or more prosaically, what avenues lupus researchers are following.

New Drugs in the Pipeline

Drugs that are in the pipeline are not difficult to find on the Internet. It takes years and vast sums of money to develop a new drug, with the hope of a matching profit only if a new blockbuster makes it to the market. So every candidate's progress is watched keenly by financial analysts as well as by the medical fraternity. However, for every drug that reaches the final stage—being tested in humans for its safety and effectiveness—nine out of ten stumble on one of the numerous hurdles along the course. Of those that reach the finishing line, break the tape, and go on sale, some may yet be withdrawn following a drug test, as rare side effects only emerge after a drug has been taken by tens of thousands of patients for a lengthy period. That is what happened with the COX-2 inhibitor Vioxx, which looked so promising for arthritis patients when first launched, but turned out to damage the hearts of some patients and was subsequently withdrawn. So the problem for drug manufacturers, doctors, patients, and authors alike is which drug in the pipeline will stay the course? And, to be honest, it's in the lap of the gods.

Here are some of those in the race for treating lupus:

Bromocriptine

This drug acts to reduce the release of a hormone called prolactin. As its name implies, prolactin encourages milk production following childbirth, but as with so many hormones, it is produced and active in both sexes. High prolactin levels, associated with tiny tumors in the pituitary gland, where it is released, lead to infertility by preventing menstruation and ovulation in young women; bromocriptine has been used to treat this condition for some years. (Novel uses for drugs that have been approved for other therapies start at an advantage because the drugs' safety has already been demonstrated in large numbers of patients.) The fact that lupus is a disease that predominantly strikes women of childbearing years has focused researchers' interest on hormones. High prolactin levels seem to stimulate the production of autoreactive antibodies in lupus, hence the idea that bringing them down with bromocriptine might help. It works in laboratory mice. Work in humans suggests that it could turn out to be on a par with hydroxychloroquine as a lupus treatment.

Prasterone

We looked at the role of hormones when considering the possible causes of lupus in Chapter 3. You first met prolactin there, and a form of androgen called dehydroepiandrosterone, or DHEA, which is a precursor of both the male hormone testosterone and the female hormones that regulate fertility in women: estradiol and progesterone. DHEA levels are often lower than average in lupus patients of both sexes, which prompted the development of a synthetic version of DHEA called prasterone (Prastera). This drug has

---

A Warning

American lupus expert Sheldon Blau alerts lupus sufferers to over-the-counter, so-called dietary supplements that profess to contain DHEA. Variously and unscientifically described as "superhormones" or "miracle drugs," they claim to promote weight loss, improve memory, fight infection, prevent cancer or heart disease, and generally to make you live forever with the body of a twenty-year-old. Be advised: They won't. Sheldon Blau speaks for medical experts everywhere when he reminds us that licensed drugs have to undergo lengthy testing for safety, purity, and effectiveness before they are let loose on the public. Supplements don't.

had a checkered career during clinical testing. In August 2005 the U.K. drug assessment authority, the National Institute for Clinical Excellence, announced that the application to approve it had been withdrawn.

Monoclonal Antibodies

We learned in Chapter 3, on the causes of lupus, that much of the damage in lupus is caused by antibodies, or B lymphocytes, that react to the body's own tissues, chiefly fragments from the interior of broken-down cells in the bloodstream. Attention has therefore been focused upon reducing the proliferation of these antibodies. On the principle of "set a thief to catch a thief," scientists have tried to design tailor-made antibodies that will seek out and destroy those elements of the immune system that promote inflammation without reducing the parts that perform a protective function. These have worked well in laboratory mice bred to exhibit lupus-like symptoms.

"Synthetic" antibodies are constructed by cloning a single antibody-producing cell, and are called *monoclonal antibodies* (MoAbs). Two MoAbs are being investigated for the treatment of lupus. One, called rituximab, was approved some years ago for the treatment of a form of cancer called non-Hodgkin's lymphoma in which B lymphocytes multiply beyond control. The MoAb attacks a marker on the surface of B lymphocytes, which grow up to produce the autoimmune antibodies, which in turn cause the inflammation that does all the harm in conditions like rheumatoid arthritis and lupus. So it seems logical to explore whether it would be effective in these conditions. In September 2004 researchers at the University of Rochester Medical Center reported that a single injection of rituximab gave eleven lupus patients, out of a total of seventeen, relief from a range of symptoms for a year or more. The improvement coincided with a drop in the number of B cells circulating in the patients' bloodstream. This was a very small trial and not randomly controlled (see Chapter 6, "Randomized Clinical Trials (RCT): The Therapeutic Gold Standard"), so judgment must be provisional.

Another monoclonal antibody currently being studied in patients with lupus or rheumatoid arthritis strikes even earlier in the antibody-producing process. Its target is a recently discovered protein that stimulates B lymphocytes, which grow up to produce the autoimmune antibodies ... and so on. A MoAb known provisionally as LymphoStat-B latches onto this B-lymphocyte stimulator (BlyS for short) and inhibits the development of harmful antibody-producing B cells. So far this particular MoAb has been shown to be side-effect free.

Selective Immunomodulators

Lupus is an autoimmune disease, but the autoimmune system plays a vital protective role in the body, so even if you could, you wouldn't want to suppress it entirely. The goal is to find a drug that will be selective: a rapier rather than a bludgeon, a drug that will remove the autoimmune antibodies causing the trouble while leaving the good antibodies to carry on with the positive work, vanquishing infection. Such drugs modify, or modulate, the immune system, hence the name immunomodulators. One such drug, code-named "LJP 394" (trade name Riquent), targets an antibody to a particular kind of DNA known as double-stranded DNA (hence its title of anti-dsDNA antibody) that shows up in the blood of lupus patients, especially when they have bouts of nephritis. So far it appears that the catchily named LJP 394 does reduce the quantity of anti-dsDNA antibodies and may also reduce the risk of nephritis.

Experimental Treatments for Kidney Damage

The most serious manifestation of lupus is kidney inflammation (nephritis). If it proves impossible to "head it off at the pass," there may come a stage when the only solution is a kidney transplant, and donor organs are in very short supply. A number of treatments short of replacement are being investigated.

A healthy body has built-in mechanisms for repairing damaged organs. One of the substances that stimulates this process has been identified and goes under another of those catchy pharmaceutical code names: BMP7. This stands for "bone *morphogenetic* (form-generating) protein number 7," and a synthetic version of it has in fact been used successfully to speed the process of recovery in broken bones. Natural BMP7 is found in the kidneys. Inflammation such as occurs in severe lupus produces scar tissue known as renal fibrosis, and researchers have discovered that BMP7 can reverse this process and stimulate the production of new, healthy tissue. So far it's only been done in laboratory mice.

Two nondrug treatments have been tried for severe or unresponsive lupus. Although not surgical, these therapies might be considered heroic. One is the use of targeted radiation, which is successful in preventing the recurrence of some cancers. A procedure called *total lymphoid irradiation (TLI)* targets the lymph nodes and other tissues where the lymphocytes—including the cells that grow up into the B cells that produce the antibodies, etc.—congregate. TLI appears to suppress some of the antibodies overproduced in lupus. It has been used successfully for some years to treat a potentially fatal form of lymphoma (cancer of the lymphatic system). Less frequently it has been tried for multiple sclerosis and rheumatoid arthritis. Its long-term safety and efficacy have not been established, and, like some drug treatments, it makes patients more susceptible to infection. It is uncertain whether it will ultimately prove useful in severe and refractory lupus, which is only infrequently life-threatening.

The other nondrug treatment is *plasmapheresis*. This is a mechanical procedure rather like kidney dialysis, in which the blood is circulated outside the body and harmful elements filtered out before the blood is returned. Plasma is the fluid in which various sorts of blood cells swim around. Pheresis (from the Greek for "removal") is the process of filtering out substances circulating in the blood. In the case of autoimmune diseases it can be used to remove some of the inflammatory antibodies and antigen-antibody complexes in the blood of lupus patients. So far it has only been used experimentally for rheumatoid arthritis, and although it removed harmful antibodies and improved some symptoms, the results are not long-lasting. It doesn't appear to provide any improvement in the kidney problems that are the most severe manifestations of lupus.

And Now for Something Completely Different

On several occasions we have commented that the human body is, by and large, if not infallibly, a self-healing organism. Self-healing is what the autoimmune system, among others, is all about. In recent years, scientists have asked whether the processes the body uses to grow and develop, as well as to heal, could be adapted to treat diseases that have so far outfoxed them. This is a step beyond making a drug in the laboratory that mimics a substance that is naturally active in the body, such as a steroid. This is using the body's own cells as a cure (see box "Chameleon Stem Cells," on the next page).

Stem cells may come from a donor, like a transplanted kidney, but preferably they are harvested from the patient's own blood. After the harvest the patient's abnormal mature cells are destroyed by use of a powerful immunosuppressant. This is the tricky stage, because at that moment, having no functional immune system, the patient is extremely vulnerable to infection. Needless to say the procedure is carried out with the patient in the hospital, in protective isolation. Once the abnormal cells are cleansed, the stem cells are reintroduced. Hopefully they mature, thrive, and produce new, normally functioning cells for the patient. This procedure is called *autologous* (self-sourced) *hematopoietic* (blood-making) stem-cell transplantation.

Used experimentally since 1997 in specially selected patients, it has been successful for some cases of another disease of the immune system, non-Hodgkin's lymphoma. It is also under consideration for rheumatoid arthritis. Because it is so risky it is only offered to patients with severe, drug-resistant, organ-threatening disease. At this moment that applies to very few lupus patients. However, it is almost certainly a form of therapy that has a very promising future.

Chameleon Stem Cells

Most adult body cells are specialists; as mature cells they are either specialist blood cells, muscle cells, brain cells, etc. They cannot switch and do a different job once they are mature. But cells start life as simpler nonspecialists known as stem cells. The most versatile stem cells are those in the embryo; they are the basis for the very beginning of life. Basic, dividing embryonic stem cells have the capacity to develop into all the different specialist cells a mature human body requires. Some embryonic stem cells are still present in the umbilical cord, and that is why the United Kingdom has set up a unit to bank cord blood harvested during birth. But even mature specialist cells, which are continually replacing themselves, start as immature forms and, in this state, can be encouraged to diversify if cleverly handled. It means harvesting immature stem cells from the site where they are produced; in the case of blood cells—white and red cells or platelets—this is in the bone marrow. Although blood cells are produced in the bone marrow, they can be harvested from blood by giving the patient something that encourages them to proliferate so that they spill out into, and can be picked up from, the bloodstream. They are then frozen in plastic bags with preservative until they are needed.

Fundamental Research in Progress

The research discussed in this chapter is mostly about potential treatments being investigated in the clinic. But what guides new treatments is fundamental research into the disease process that goes on in laboratories, behind the scenes. Several studies are looking at ways of reducing the number of autoimmune B cells produced in lupus, and similar diseases, and also looking at understanding how they are different from B cells in people without lupus. Studies are also going on to identify the genes that make people susceptible to lupus and other autoimmune diseases.

Dr. Madeleine Devey, of the Arthritis Research Campaign (ARC), believes that understanding genetics will eventually lead to much better targeted treatment for lupus. She says, "Therapy has improved markedly in recent years, and the death rate of this potentially fatal condition has fallen. In the U.K., at Imperial College, London, they are making a big effort to understand the genetics of lupus in mice, with the strong likelihood that these genes will have exact counterparts in humans."

Meanwhile, in the U.S., researchers at the University of Minnesota recently announced that they have identified the first gene variant to be associated with lupus. Although it is found in approximately 16 percent of unaffected Caucasians, it is present in nearly 25 percent of those with lupus or insulin-dependent diabetes, another autoimmune condition. Timothy Behrens, the principal investigator, says, "This is the first time we have identified a variant that predisposes [a person] to many different autoimmune diseases." Behrens believes that dozens of genes may well turn out to be responsible for lupus and that discovering the combination of these genes will be important to developing better diagnosis and treatment of the disease.

In Closing

At first, a diagnosis of lupus may seem like a death sentence. But I hope that in reading this book you have realized that there is a worthwhile life after the bad news. If you work with the professionals and adopt a proactive approach to managing your particular lupus the beast can be tamed. And your self-esteem will be increased in the process.

Glossary

allergic: showing an unhealthy response to something as a result of previous exposure

alphafetoprotein (AFP): protein produced in the fetus's liver, and picked up in the mother's blood, which reveals information on fetal development

androgen: a general term for male sex hormone; testosterone is the principal male sex hormone

anemia: shortage of oxygen-carrying red cells in the blood

angiotensin converting enzyme (ACE) inhibitor: blood-pressure-lowering drug

ankylosing spondylitis: form of arthritis that affects the vertebrae

antibody: disease-fighting cell produced in response to a specific antigen

anticardiolipin: antibody associated with blood-clotting problems

anticoagulant: drug that reduces a tendency for the blood to clot

antigen: something that prompts antibody reaction

antinuclear antibody (ANA): antibody that reacts to material from the cell nucleus often present in connective tissue diseases

antioxidant: molecule able to counteract the damaging effects of free oxygen atoms (free radicals) on the body

antiphospholipid antibody syndrome (APS): also Hughes' syndrome; a condition causing clots inside blood vessels and predisposing women to miscarriage

apoptosis: programmed cell death

arrhythmia: uneven heartbeat; an early sign of cardiovascular disease

arthritis: inflammation of joints accompanied by pain and swelling; has many varieties

aura: visual disturbance that sometimes precedes migraine or seizure; consists of flashing lights, bright or blind spots, blurred vision

autoimmune disease: condition in which cells of the immune system (antibodies) attack the body's own tissues *autologous:* originating with the self; e.g., harvesting the patient's own blood or stem cells

autoreactive: acting against the body's own tissues; used to describe antibodies

avascular necrosis: bone or tendon damage caused by reduced blood supply

bisphosphonate: antiosteoporosis drug

B lymphocytes: lymphocytes that produce antibodies; see T lymphocytes

calcium antagonist: blood-pressure-lowering drug that acts on blood-vessel walls

casein: one of the proteins in cheese

chronic: describes a condition that comes and goes; opposite of acute

clusters: incidence of disease concentrated in one geographic location

cognitive behavioral therapy (CBT): changing how someone thinks and evaluates events

colonoscopy: internal investigation of the colon (large bowel) with fiber-optic camera

comparator: standard treatment or drug against which a new drug is assessed

complement: collections of proteins that support antibody activity

compliance: following medical instructions; opposite of noncompliance

concordant: having a characteristic in common; matching

connective tissue disease (CTD): group of diseases (including lupus) that affect related tissues widely distributed throughout the body

core decompression: surgical treatment for bone necrosis designed to stimulate healthy cell growth

corticosteroid, cortisone: powerful anti-inflammatory drug modeled on a naturally occurring human hormone, cortisol

cyclooxygenase (COX): enzyme that stimulates the production of prostaglandins; painkillers that inhibit COX-2 selectively cause fewer gastric side effects

cytokines: chemical messengers that communicate between cells

dehydroepiandrosterone (DHEA): precursor to the sex hormones testosterone in men and estradiol and progesterone in women; often below normal in lupus patients

deoxyribonucleic acid (DNA): material in genes that transmits hereditary information

differential diagnosis: evaluating a number of diagnoses and selecting the most likely

diuretic: drug that increases fluid excretion and helps lower blood pressure

echocardiograph: graphic representation of the interior of the heart using sound waves

E. coli: common bacteria (names of genus and species are usually printed in Latin and italic)

edema: accumulation of fluid in tissue spaces

electrocardiogram: graph of the electric impulses that regulate the heart

endocarditis: inflammation of the lining of the heart

endorphins: chemicals produced in the brain that reduce pain and increase a sense of well-being

epidemiology: study of disease in populations

erythema nodosum: form of blood-vessel inflammation (vasculitis) characterized by painful, reddish nodules

erythrocyte: red blood cell

erythrocyte sedimentation rate (ESR): speed at which red blood cells in solution sink to the bottom of a test tube; indicator of unspecified infection or inflammation

estrogen: one of the hormones regulating the female menstrual cycle

fibromyalgia: rheumatic syndrome characterized by generalized muscle pain and fatigue

genome: total information for a living system contained in DNA sequences

hematologist: specialist in blood disorders

hematopoietic: producing blood cells

hemophilia: inherited, sex-linked, potentially fatal bleeding disorder caused by absence of blood-clotting factors; women carry it, men suffer it

heart-block: heartbeat irregularities due to misfiring of electrical signals in the heart

herpesviruses: group of common viruses (chickenpox, cold sores, shingles) that, once caught, often recur; suspected of involvement in autoimmune diseases

iatrogenic: caused by doctors or medical treatment

immune complex: "clumps" of warring antibody/antigen that cause damage to surrounding tissue

incidence: number of new cases of a disease

leukemia: cancer of blood-producing tissue leading to overproduction of abnormal white-cell forms and a reduction of normal blood cells

lipids: soluble fats circulating in the blood; high levels are associated with stroke and heart attack; cholesterol is a lipid

lymphocyte: white cell active in the immune system

macular retinopathy: damage caused by pigment deposited in the retina, the part of the eye that forms and relays images to the brain

magnetic resonance imaging (MRI): diagnostic technique using radio-frequency pulses to create three-dimensional images of body tissues

major histocompatibility complex (MHC): genes that code for which tissue types the body recognizes as compatible and which are rejected as foreign

malar rash: so-called butterfly rash, usually facial, characteristic of lupus

metabolize/metabolism: biological process by which energy is extracted from oxygen and nutrients and waste products eliminated

monoclonal antibodies (MoAbs): synthetic antibodies targeted on a single antigen

morphogenetic: form-generating; stimulating growth of new tissue

myalgic encephalitis (ME): another name for chronic fatigue syndrome; see fibromyalgia, which some experts recognize as the same illness

necrosis: tissue damage through erosion, decay, or rupture

neonatal: immediately after birth

nephritis: inflammation of the kidneys

nephrologist: specialist in kidney disease

neural-tube defect (NTD): damage to the fetal brain or spinal cord

noncompliance: see compliance

ophthalmologist: specialist in eye disease

opiates: group of powerful painkillers (e.g., morphine)

osteoarthritis: joint pain and deformity caused by wear and tear

osteonecrosis: bone-cell decay or "death"

osteoporosis: loss of bone density leading to brittle bone and easy fracture

patellar tendon: tendon tethering the quadriceps muscle at the front of the knee and maintaining the stability of the joint upon which the kneecap (patella) is set

pericarditis: inflammation of the membrane surrounding the heart

pericardium: outer membrane surrounding the heart

photosensitive: abnormal or extreme reaction to light

placebo: dummy pill used in clinical trials to compare the effectiveness of an active drug

placebo effect: improvement demonstrated by patients who have been administered a dummy pill

plasmapheresis: filtering blood outside the body to remove abnormal cells

platelet: blood cell that initiates clotting; also thrombocyte (clotting cell)

pleura: membrane surrounding the lungs

pleurisy: inflammation of the membrane surrounding the lungs

polymyositis, dermatomyositis (PM-DM): form of CTD, often occurring together, characterized by generalized muscle and skin inflammation

preeclampsia: failure of the kidneys to filter waste products from the body during the last phase of pregnancy

prevalence: total number of those with a condition in a given population

prognosis: predicted outcome of a disease or treatment

prostaglandin: substance that contributes to, and modifies, inflammation and blood clotting

prostaglandin inhibitor: drug that inhibits the activity of prostaglandins (e.g., aspirin and NSAIDs)

psoralen: chemical found in some plants that increases photosensitivity

pulmonary emboli: fragments of blood clots that obstruct the lungs

pulse therapy: administering a drug in "bursts" via intravenous injection

randomized, controlled trial (RCT): drug test in which patients are randomly assigned to either an active or a comparator (usually standard) treatment

randomized, placebo-controlled, double-blind trial: drug test in which treatment is tested against a patient group taking a dummy pill, and neither patients nor administering physicians know which is which

Raynaud's phenomenon or *syndrome:* condition characterized by numb, blue fingers and toes, caused by vasospasm in response to cold or other stimuli

rheumatoid arthritis: inflammatory CTD principally affecting multidirectional (synovial) joints, also blood vessels and membranes

rheumatoid factor: antibody found in the blood of about 80 percent of rheumatoid arthritis patients and some with other inflammatory conditions

rheumatologist: specialist in inflammatory conditions

ribonucleic acid (RNA): building-block chemicals that transfer genetic information from DNA; unlike DNA, RNA can leave the nucleus of a cell

salmonella: group of germs (bacilli) associated with food poisoning in humans

sclerosis, scleroderma: hardening of connective tissue or skin

sicca syndrome: dry eyes and mouth caused by blockage of fluid-secreting ducts by inflammation; see also Sjögren's syndrome

Sjögren's syndrome: autoimmune disease that reduces the secretions of many glands of the body, resulting in severe dryness of the eyes, mouth, and vagina

statin: lipid-lowering drug that has other beneficial side effects

systemic: affecting organs throughout the body

systemic lupus erythematosus (SLE): full name and acronym of lupus

therapeutics: science of treating illness with drugs

thrombocyte: cell that promotes clotting; see platelet

thrombophlebitis: inflammation of veins, often in legs

tinnitus: persistent ringing in the ears

T lymphocytes (also B lymphocytes): subclasses of lymphocytes with different functions in the immune process

total lymphoid irradiation (TLI): irradiation of lymph nodes with aim of reducing abnormal lymphocytes that congregate there

vasculitis: inflammation of blood vessels

vasoconstrictors: drugs that cause blood vessels to constrict

vasospasm: spasmodic contraction, closing down of small blood vessels

vesicles: small bladder-like cavities

Further Reading

Aladjem, Henrietta (founder of the Lupus Foundation of America). *The Challenges of Lupus: Insights and Hope.* New York: Avery, 1998.

Blau, Sheldon Paul, and Dodi Schultz. *Living with Lupus: The Complete Guide,* 2d rev. ed. Cambridge, MA: Da Capo Press, 2004.

Berne, Katrina. *Chronic Fatigue Syndrome, Fibromyalgia and Other Invisible Illnesses,* 3d ed. Alameda, CA: Hunter House Publishers, 2002.

Holden, Triona. *Positive Options for Living with Antiphospholipid Syndrome (APS).* Alameda, CA: Hunter House Publishers, 2003.

Holden, Triona, and Graham Hughes. *Talking about Lupus: What to Do and How to Cope.* London: Piatkus Books, 2004.

Hughes, Graham. *Lupus: The Facts.* Oxford, U.K.: Oxford University Press, 2000.

Lahita, Robert G., and Robert H. Phillips. *Lupus Q&A: Everything You Need to Know,* rev. ed. New York: Avery, 2004.

Phillips, Robert H. *Coping with Lupus,* 3d ed. New York: Avery, 2001.

Pratt, Maureen, David Hallegua, and Daniel J. Wallace. *Taking Charge of Lupus: How to Manage the Disease and Make the Most of Your Life.* New York: New American Library, 2002.

Wallace, Daniel J. *The Lupus Book: A Guide for Patients and Their Families,* 3rd ed. Oxford, U.K.: Oxford University Press, 2005.

▶ ▶ ▶

The following publications are available from Lupus U.K. (www.lupusuk.com; see Resources):

Butterfly Traveller, ELEF and Novartis Pharma Verlag, 2000. A medical phrasebook for the lupus patient and other travelers, in twelve different languages.

Lupus: A GP Guide to Diagnosis, Lupus U.K., 2000.

Living with Lupus (video), Lupus U.K. A guide for patients.

Resources

Lupus Research and Support Organizations

Patient-support organizations for lupus exist all over the world. National associations will usually put you in touch with local groups, or, if you search the Internet, you may be able to locate them directly. In addition to patient support, some organizations focus on research. Their scope may be broader than lupus and embrace other forms of inflammatory arthritis, connective tissue diseases, or autoimmune diseases. Here are two of the most prominent lupus-related organizations in the United States:

Arthritis Foundation
P.O. Box 7669
Atlanta GA 30357-0669
(800) 568-4045
(404) 872-7100
Website: www.arthritis.org
Their website, which covers all forms of arthritis, provides information, news stories, the latest research, patient histories, and details of local offices all over the country.

Lupus Foundation of America
2000 L Street NW, Suite 710
Washington DC 20036
(202) 349-1156
Website: www.lupus.org
An organization with many offerings: patient support and chat rooms, news, information, advice and patient contact networks, clinical trials recruiting, a reading list. The scope is seemingly endless.

Lupus Organizations in Other Countries

Australia

Lupus Australia Foundation
Level 2, 247–251 Flinders Ln.
Melbourne VIC 3000, Australia
Phone: +61-3-9650-5348
Website: www.lupusvic.org.au
A number of linked Australian state lupus-support organizations are at this Melbourne address.

Canada

Lupus Canada
590 Alden Rd., Suite 211
Markham ON L3R 8N2, Canada
(800) 661-1468 (in Canada)
(905) 313-0004
E-mail: lupuscanada@bellnet.ca
Website: www.lupuscanada.org
A number of Canadian provinces' lupus organizations are listed on the website. The Lupus Society of Alberta website (www.lupus.ab.ca) features a wonderful animated cartoon that explains lupus antibody behavior and makes you laugh!

Europe

The Arthritis Research Campaign (ARC)
Copeman House
St. Mary's Ct. ,St. Mary's Gate
Chesterfield Derbyshire S41 7TD, England
Phone: +44-870-850-5000
Website: www.arc.org.uk
ARC's website provides details of research centers and scientific information about all forms of arthritis. ARC also publishes leaflets and a magazine called *Arthritis Today*.

Hughes' Syndrome Foundation
The Rayne Institute, Louise Coote Lupus Unit
Gassiot House
St. Thomas' Hospital
London SE1 7EH, England
Phone: +44-20-7188-8217

+44-20-7188-7188, ext. 83570
Website: www.hughes-syndrome.org
The Louise Coote Lupus Centre is based at The Rayne Institute at St.
Thomas' Hospital. The Institute (one of several) was established by the
charitable Rayne Foundation with a mission to facilitate the flow of
ideas between medical research and practicing doctors.

LUPUS UK
St James House
Eastern Rd.
Romford Essex RM1 3NH, England
Phone: +44-1708-731251
Website: www.lupusuk.com
A comprehensive site with news, information, advice, support contacts,
and details of research in progress.

European Lupus Erythematosus Federation (ELEF)
St. James House
Eastern Rd.
Romford Essex RM1 3NH, England
Phone: +44-1708-731251
Website: www.elef.rheumanet.org

Other Helpful Organizations and Websites

A large number of associations and organizations in the United States
present themselves instantly with an Internet search. I've listed below
some of those I found most helpful (and entertaining):

Organizations
The American Autoimmune Related Diseases Association
www.aarda.org

National Institute of Arthritis, Musculoskeletal, and Skin Diseases
www.niams.nih.gov

Websites
Alexandra Y. Zhang, M.D., and Craig E. Elmets, M.D. "Drug-Induced
Photosensitivity." www.emedicine.com/derm/topic108.htm (advice on
things that increase photosensitivity).

Kevin J. McElwee. "Immunology"
www.keratin.com/am/amindex.shtml (a history of the immune system).

Lupus Society of Alberta (Canada). "What Is Lupus? An Animated Explanation" http://www.lupus.ab.ca/viewpage.asp?p=resources-flash (animated cartoon on what happens in lupus—amuses and informs).

Quackwatch: Your Guide to Quackery, Health Fraud, and Intelligent Decisions. www.quackwatch.org (information about fraud, scams, alerts about unsubstantiated medical claims)

Tips on Internet Searching

The Internet is a source of such endless information that the only problem is sorting the good information from the bad. Some useful tips: The boxes at the side of the page are paid for, so their sponsors (who are advertisers) may have an axe to grind. The suffix ".org" implies a charity or an organization whose primary focus is not commercial. The suffix ".edu" implies an academic or educational site, likely to be well informed but possibly narrow or esoteric in focus. Beware of jazzy, all-singing, all-dancing sites. They probably aren't serious. If you haven't yet found the impressive search engine Google, try it (www.google.com).

If you don't have online access at home, go to the public library and browse for free. Information, support, and the experience of other people with lupus are all waiting out there to be shared.

Index

More Hunter House Books

POSITIVE OPTIONS FOR SJÖGREN'S SYNDROME: Self-Help and Treatment
by Sue Dyson

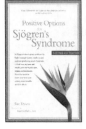

In Sjögren's ("show-grins") syndrome the body's immune system attacks its own moisture-producing glands. Symptoms include dry eyes and mouth, joint, and muscle pain, difficulty in swallowing, fatigue, and depression. Nine out of ten sufferers are women. Author Sue Dyson has Sjögren's, and she evaluates a full range of self-help and treatment options, mainstream and alternative, giving their possible benefits and side effects.

128 pages ... Paperback $12.95

POSITIVE OPTIONS FOR REFLEX SYMPATHETIC DYSTROPHY (RSD): Self-Help and Treatment *by Elena Juris*

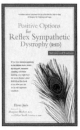

RSD, also called Complex Regional Pain Syndrome, is characterized by severe nerve pain, swelling, and extreme sensitivity to touch. Simple conditions such as sprains can escalate into RSD. There is no known cure, but with prompt treatment many people go into remission or experience reduced symptoms. This book offers medical information and practical advice and also covers complementary therapies.

224 pages ... Paperback $14.95

THE JOURNEY TO PAIN RELIEF: A Hands-On Guide to Breakthroughs in Pain Treatment *by Phyllis Berger*

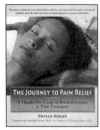

Written for pain sufferers *and* professionals, this book describes new techniques for blocking pain pathways with low-voltage electrical currents and acupuncture, all discussed and illustrated in detail. Other sections outline self-help options including how to increase pain-free movements with carefully selected exercise.

264 pages ... Paperback $18.95

THE ART OF GETTING WELL: A Five-Step Plan for Maximizing Health When You Have a Chronic Illness
by David Spero, R.N.

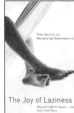

Written for people dealing with chronic illness, this is a five-step program for optimizing your energy and health: Slow down, save energy for the things that matter — make small, progressive changes — get help and nourish social ties — value your body, treat it with respect — take responsibility for getting the best care you can.

224 pages ... Paperback $16.95

THE JOY OF LAZINESS: Why Life is Better Slower — and How to Get There *by Peter Axt, Ph.D., and Michaela Axt-Gadermann, M.D.*

The early bird may get the worm, but late sleepers live longer. The authors show why being "lazy" can make your immune system stronger, too much exercise can make you sick, fasting delays aging, and being relaxed makes you smarter and healthier. They show how to conserve energy and monitor your stress level, and outline an exercise program to promote both fitness and a long life.

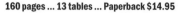

160 pages ... 13 tables ... Paperback $14.95